To the memory of George Oral Waring III, M.D. (1941–2015):
mentor, friend, and lebenskünstler.

Contents

Acknowledgments vii

Preface ix

1 Why You Need Glasses or Contacts 1

2 Vision Correction Surgery: An Overview . . 15

3 Are You a Candidate for
Vision Correction Surgery? 27

4 The Preoperative Evaluation 32

5 LASIK 37

6 PRK 65

7 Implantable Contact Lens 83

8 Refractive Lens Exchange 95

9 Choosing an Eye Surgeon 110

In Closing 123

Resources 125

Glossary 129

Index 141

About the Authors 151

Acknowledgments

I'm grateful to my father, who taught me to be uncompromising in the pursuit of excellence, and my mother, who taught me that great relationships require compromise. I'm particularly grateful to my fabulous wife, Nicole, for her patience with the demands of my chosen career. at times, she must wish that I had listened more to my mother's advice.

Robert K. Maloney, M.D.

I wish to thank my husband and my daughters, without whose support I could not nurture my love of my chosen field while keeping a work-life harmony that together bring color and fulfillment to my days.

Neda Shamie, M.D.

Preface

Because you have opened this book, you probably don't see as well as you'd like. And perhaps you dislike wearing glasses or contact lenses. Maybe you love being active, and your glasses are an inconvenience when you exercise vigorously. Perhaps you love the water, but your contacts wash out when you open your eyes.

Are you tired of your glasses fogging up when you open the dishwasher or when you come inside on a cold day? Do you want to be a policeman, a fireman, or a Navy SEAL, but you cannot even be considered because of your poor vision? Maybe you don't like the way you look in glasses. Whatever your personal story is, you're seeking a way to achieve better vision without glasses or contact lenses.

From my own experience, I have a pretty good idea how you feel. I was nearsighted for twenty-six years. I hated wearing glasses because of their appearance and my limited peripheral vision. Contacts were tolerable, but I disliked the inconvenience of caring for them, and carrying around all the paraphernalia I needed to maintain them. Mostly, I hated being blind. I wanted the freedom of opening my eyes in the morning and seeing perfectly all day long. I became a specialist in vision correction surgery largely because I disliked my own poor vision and wanted something better. Then, in 1996, I had the LASIK procedure, and I've had perfect vision ever since.

Some eye doctors discourage people from considering LASIK and other vision correction procedures. They say you shouldn't consider vision correction surgery if you can wear glasses or contacts. I disagree. To me, that is like telling a man with a bad knee on crutches that he shouldn't get the ligaments in his knee repaired. If your eyes aren't functioning properly, modern medicine offers the technology to fix your eyes safely. You shouldn't have to continue depending on glasses or contacts.

When I started doing vision correction surgery more than twenty years ago, the technology and procedures were relatively primitive. My colleagues and I who were pioneering this field had relatively modest goals for our patients: we hoped to get the majority of people seeing pretty well without glasses. When our patients needed perfect vision after surgery, we expected they would still wear glasses.

It was a pleasant surprise when a patient got 20/20 vision. However, with advances in technology and surgical techniques, the results we get today with vision correction surgery have completely changed. Our expectation now is that almost everyone who has vision correction surgery will be able to see 20/20 without glasses. The only exception is that some patients might need reading glasses; otherwise, almost everyone who undergoes vision correction surgery won't even own a pair of glasses anymore. In fact, the majority of our patients now see better than 20/20—a result we refer to as "super vision" or "supranormal vision."

This brings me to the first theme of this book: if you are like most people, you can get rid of your glasses safely and permanently. There are a variety of surgical procedures that can enable you to get rid of your glasses; these include procedures such as LASIK, PRK, refractive lens exchange, and contact lens implants. With the right procedure, you can wake up in the morning with clear vision every day. You can open the medicine cabinet and scoop all the contact lens solutions directly into the trash can. You can lose your glasses…on purpose.

I should note, however, that not everyone should have vision correction surgery. Some people have medical conditions that disqualify them. Others have needs or expectations that simply can't be met by today's surgical procedures. Also, although these procedures are remarkably safe, there are risks, such as night-vision disturbances. These risks need to be balanced against the benefits of surgery in each person individually.

Preface

The second theme of the book is that even though vision correction surgery is a modern miracle, the decision to have it should be made carefully, and you need to choose a vision correction procedure that is uniquely customized for you. Every pair of eyes is different. What is right for one person is not right for another. Most people want optimal distance vision, but for others, close-up vision for reading is more important.

If you are contemplating vision correction surgery, you will want to explore which procedure is best for your eyes, your needs, and your overall health. I encourage you to learn exactly what is involved in a procedure, find out what results you can expect, and also learn about all the possible risks and complications. Finally, make sure you choose an experienced, qualified surgeon—someone you can really trust.

We wrote this book to provide you with an easy-to-understand educational tool that will answer your questions about today's most popular vision correction surgical procedures, including LASIK, implantable contact lenses, and everything in between. We hope you'll find it helpful.

Robert K. Maloney, M.D.

Why You Need Glasses or Contacts

Sight is our most precious sense. Our eyes enable us to take in the surrounding world. Without sight, the way we perceive the world would be forever changed. No wonder the eyes are often elevated in literature, art, religion, and philosophy to symbolize everything from the windows of the soul to supreme wisdom. Indeed, the eyes are a marvel of mechanics, performing many complicated functions in a very short time—in the blink of an eye, you might say.

However, changes within the eyeball may occur, resulting in impaired vision. Objects that we once viewed with crystal clarity may become blurred or distorted. To better understand how vision may change, let's first examine how vision normally happens.

How Vision Happens

You may have heard the comparison between a camera and the human eye. Just as a camera takes in light and transforms it into an image on film, your eye does virtually the same thing, only the "film" is your retina and your brain "develops" the image. We see objects when light, which is reflected by the objects, passes through the front layers of the eye and strikes the retina, at the back of the eye. Our brain then interprets the shapes, colors, and dimensions of the objects we see.

A clearly focused object is the result of normal vision. However, just as an improper focus of light entering a camera lens will blur a photo, if light entering the eyeball does not focus properly on the retina, the result is blurred vision.

How the Eye Sees

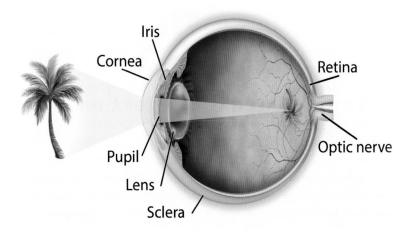

Figure 1. Light from an object, such as a palm tree, is focused by the cornea and lens onto the retina. The retina turns the light into electrical signals that travel through the optic nerve to the brain, which identifies the object.

It is helpful to think of seeing as six distinct steps, outlined below, which are roughly similar to the way a camera processes an image *(Figure 1)*.

Light Reflects Off an Object

Suppose you are on a tropical beach, looking at a palm tree as its fronds wave in the ocean breeze. You're actually seeing the light from the sun reflecting off the leaves. That is why you can't see in the dark: there is no light present to reflect off objects and enter your eye.

Light Enters the Eye through the Cornea

The light reflected from the leaves reaches your eye. It first enters the *cornea.* The cornea is the part of your eye you touch when you put in a contact lens. It is a transparent dome, the size of a dime and as thick as a credit card. The cornea provides most of the eye's focusing power, so small changes in its curvature can make an enormous difference in how clearly you see objects. The curved surface of the cornea bends the incoming light so that the rays converge, instead of remaining parallel as they enter the eye. Thus, the cornea does the initial focusing work of the eye.

2

Light Passes through the Pupil

After passing through the cornea, the light reaches the *pupil*. The pupil is a hole in the *iris,* which is a thin layer of tissue in the middle of the eye. Muscles in the iris constrict or dilate the pupil to let the optimal amount of light pass through into the eye's interior, just like the f-stop in a camera.

Light Is Focused by the Lens

The light that passes through the pupil then enters the *lens* of the eye. The lens is behind the iris. In a healthy, young eye, the lens rapidly adjusts its focus for distance or near vision. The lens provides the final focus to create a clear image for the retina.

Light Reaches the Retina

The light reaches the back of the eye, where the *retina* lies. If you have normal vision, there is a clear image of the palm tree on the retina. The retina's photoreceptor cells, the rods and cones, convert the image of the tree to signals that the brain can understand.

Light Signals Are Interpreted by the Brain

Finally, the signals are carried to the brain through the nerve bundle at the back of the eye—the *optic nerve,* which consists of millions of nerve fibers. The brain receives and interprets the signals, and it is at that point that you actually see.

Refractive Errors:
Nearsightedness, Farsightedness, and Astigmatism

The eye is a marvelous, but complicated, part of our bodies. As you age, a variety of problems with vision may arise. These problems fall into two classes: problems that can be corrected with glasses or contacts and problems that can't be. If your vision can be corrected with glasses and contacts, your problem is called a *refractive error,* and we can usually get rid of your glasses and contacts with the appropriate surgical procedure. Refractive errors are focusing problems in the eye. If glasses and contacts don't correct your vision, you have a bigger problem, and you may need a different kind of surgery, such as cataract surgery.

If you have cataracts, you might want to consult our book, *Cataract Surgery: A Patient's Guide to Cataract Treatment.*

Normal Vision

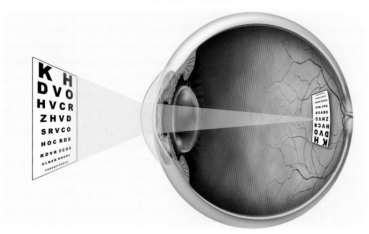

Figure 2. Light from an object comes to a perfect focus on the retina.

The book you are reading now is mainly concerned with the first class of problems, refractive errors, and how to correct them permanently.

How well you see is determined, for the most part, by how accurately your eyes are able to focus, or *refract,* light. In a normal eye, the light that enters the eye is refracted to a precise point on the retina *(Figure 2).* Unfortunately, this precise focus often does not occur. The result is various forms of blurry vision due to refractive error. If you have a refractive error, you need glasses or contacts to see clearly. There are two basic types of refractive error: *myopia* and *hyperopia.* Each of these can occur alone or in combination with astigmatism.

Myopia (Nearsightedness)

Also known as *nearsightedness,* myopia is a condition in which you can see nearby objects clearly, but objects at a distance appear blurred. This happens when light reflecting from a faraway object enters the eye and comes to a point of focus too soon, before it reaches the retina *(Figure 3).* Myopia may be due to any one of three causes. First, the cornea may have too much curvature, which causes the light to bend too much and focus in front of the retina. Second, the lens may be too strong, again focusing the light too quickly so the focus occurs before the retina. Third, the eyeball may be too long—

Nearsighted Vision (Myopia)

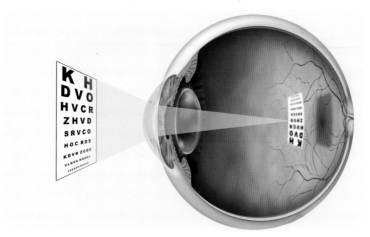

Figure 3. The focusing power of the cornea and lens is too strong, so light from an object is focused in front of the retina. The result is blurry vision.

the retina is too far back for the combined focusing power of the cornea and lens. Each of these three possible causes of myopia results in light coming to focus in front of the retina.

In general terms, nearsightedness can be corrected surgically in two ways: either move the retina forward toward the front of the eye, or move the focus of light back toward the retina. The retina can be moved forward by resecting a strip of sclera around the equator of the eye and sewing the remaining front and back halves of the eye back together. This operation was invented in Russia and is risky, so it has never been done in the United States (fortunately).

The other method is to reduce the focusing power of the front part of the eye so that the focus of light moves back to the proper spot on the retina. The focusing power of the front part of the eye can be reduced in a few ways. We can reduce the power of the cornea by flattening it out. This is how LASIK and PRK surgeries correct nearsightedness. Another option is to replace the lens of the eye with a synthetic lens that has less focusing power, a procedure called *refractive lens exchange (RLE)*. A third option is to insert a tiny contact lens in front of the natural lens to subtract focusing power. This is called an *implantable contact lens (ICL)* and is suitable for highly nearsighted people.

Farsighted Vision (Hyperopia)

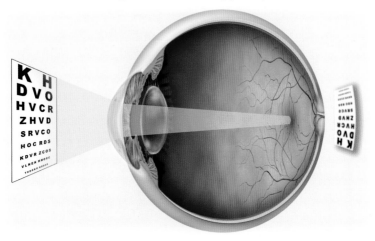

Figure 4. The focusing power of the cornea and lens is too weak. Light from an object is focused behind the retina, causing blurry vision.

Hyperopia (Farsightedness)

People with hyperopia, or *farsightedness,* see close objects blurry when they are young. As they age, distant objects get blurry, too, but not as blurry as close objects. In hyperopia, the light rays coming into the eye are not bent sharply enough, and are focused behind, rather than on, the retina. The result is a blurred image *(Figure 4)*. Like myopia, there are three possible causes for hyperopia. First, the cornea may not have enough curvature, which causes the light to bend too little and focus behind the retina. Second, the lens may be too weak, again focusing the light too weakly, so the focus occurs behind the retina. Third, the eyeball can be too short—the retina is too close for the combined focusing power of the cornea and lens.

Because the lens is very elastic in youth, younger people who are mildly hyperopic can often compensate for it by using the focusing muscles around the lens to fine-tune the focus by bending light more steeply. This action brings the point of focus forward toward the retina, allowing them to see more clearly. However, because the muscles weaken and the lens becomes less pliable as we age, these individuals eventually lose that ability and may no longer see well at a distance or close up. After age forty, they may be completely dependent on eyeglasses or contact lenses for both close and distant vision.

Farsightedness can be corrected surgically in ways similar to nearsightedness. The focusing power of the cornea can be increased with LASIK or PRK, so that the focus of light moves forward onto the retina. Refractive lens exchange, in which the natural lens is replaced with a stronger synthetic lens, is often an excellent option. The new lens can be multifocal, which restores both distance and reading vision.

Astigmatism

Many individuals with myopia or hyperopia also have some degree of *astigmatism.* People with significant astigmatism experience blurred or distorted vision at all distances. Astigmatism means that your cornea, instead of being spherical like a basketball, is slightly oval, shaped more like the side of a football. As a result, light rays entering the eye from different points on the cornea's surface are bent differently and are focused at several different points rather than meeting at just one focal point. Astigmatism can also result if the lens of the eye is oval instead of round.

Astigmatism, by itself or in combination with nearsightedness or farsightedness, can be corrected with LASIK or PRK. To correct astigmatism with LASIK or PRK, the laser removes an oval-shaped area of tissue instead of a round shape. Astigmatism can also be corrected by making tiny incisions at the periphery of the cornea. These are called *relaxing incisions,* because they allow the oval cornea to relax outward and become spherical. Astigmatism can also be corrected with refractive lens exchange or an implantable contact lens by implanting a lens that has built-in astigmatism correction. These lenses are called *toric* lenses.

Presbyopia, or Why You Need Reading Glasses

It is altogether normal that we need reading glasses as we age. Even if you have enjoyed perfect vision your whole life, you will need reading glasses in your mid-forties. Guaranteed. It happens to every human being. It even happens to primates like apes and gorillas. The loss of reading vision with age is called *presbyopia,* which is Latin for "old eyes."

How the Lens Focuses

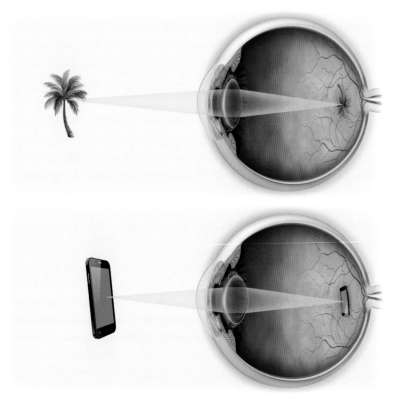

Figure 5. The lens in the eye changes its shape to allow you to focus on far and close objects. When the lens is relaxed, the normal eye is focused for distance (top illustration) and light rays from an object focus sharply on the retina. To see up close, the muscle that controls the lens contracts, changing the shape of the lens. This focuses the eye for close vision.

If you've had good distance vision, you'll notice at around age forty-five that you need to hold things farther away to read. The old joke is that your arms have gotten shorter. You can no longer read the menu or your cell phone. Most people get reading glasses at this point. If you have worn contacts or glasses, in your mid-forties you find that you need contacts plus reading glasses, or you need bifocal glasses. All of a sudden, the hassles with your vision have doubled. This section explains why this happens and what we can do about it.

Causes of Presbyopia

As we explained earlier, the eye is similar to a camera. When you take a photo of an object far away, and then you take a photo of something up close, the camera must change its focus for the close shot. In the old days, the photographer would rotate the lens to refocus the camera. Nowadays, autofocus cameras refocus the camera automatically. Even with the autofocus feature, there is still focusing taking place; if you listen, you can hear the lens move as you point the camera at different scenes.

The eye works the same way. The natural lens of the eye does the focusing. When you look at something far away, the brain signals the muscle that changes the focusing power of the eye's lens to relax, which focuses the eye for distance. To look at something up close, the brain tells the muscle to contract, focusing the eye for close vision *(Figure 5)*. All day long, in the normal youthful eye, the lens is constantly changing its focus, without thought or awareness, to allow a person to see things both close and far away.

As we age, the natural lens gradually hardens and loses its ability to change its focus. The lens in effect becomes stuck on a single focus. It's as if the autofocus on your camera got stuck on distance focus. You can take photos of mountains and baseball games just fine, but photos of someone's face across the table are blurry. It is important to note that, unless you are farsighted, presbyopia doesn't impair your distance vision. Your natural lens gets stuck on the distance setting, so your distance vision doesn't change. The lens's ability to change the focus for close up is what is lost. Your distance vision normally stays good, but you need reading glasses to see close.

The surgical correction of presbyopia is a complicated subject and will be discussed in detail in a later chapter.

Range of Vision

So far, we have been talking about distance and near vision. We need to be a little more precise *(Figures 6 to 8)*. When we eye surgeons assess your visual needs after surgery, we think in terms of what you need at each of three ranges of vision: distance, near, and intermediate.

Nonmedical people think of *distance vision* as applying to things farther than about twenty feet away. Eye doctors

Ranges of Vision

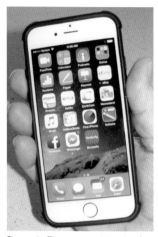

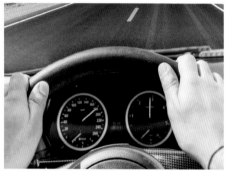

Figure 7. Intermediate vision refers to viewing objects at finger-tip range—items such as a computer screen or the dashboard of your car.

Figure 6. Close range vision involves viewing items close-up—such as newspapers, menus, and your cell phone.

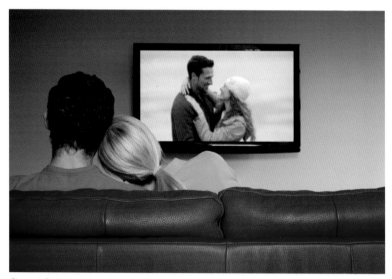

Figure 8. Distance range vision involves objects viewed beyond your fingertips; this includes such things as road signs, a television screen, or someone sitting across from you at a table.

think of distance vision as seeing anything farther away than the fingertips of your outstretched hand. Even as a person ages and requires glasses for close vision, she normally can still see things beyond her fingertips clearly. Distance vision is used to drive, play sports, watch television, and see faces across a dinner table.

Near vision is used for seeing things at the distance you would hold a book, about fourteen inches away. Near vision is used for seeing your cell phone, reading a menu, threading a needle, and putting on makeup.

There is another important range of vision, called *intermediate vision,* which is in between distance and near vision. Intermediate vision is used for seeing things at fingertip distance on your outstretched hand, like a computer screen, the prices on the shelves in the supermarket, or the speedometer on your car.

Distance, intermediate, and near vision are all important for optimal vision. As a person ages, he first loses near vision, usually around age forty-five, and needs to get reading glasses. He can still see intermediate objects like his computer screen. The lens in his eye continues to harden with age, losing more of its focusing ability. Around age fifty-two, intermediate vision gets blurry and he needs to get glasses for computer use, too.

Presbyopia and Nearsightedness

Earlier paragraphs describe what happens to people with perfect distance vision as they age. Maybe you didn't have perfect distance vision to begin with. Likely, you were myopic. Being nearsighted, you never could see well far away, but you always could read without glasses. So what happens to you as you age? After the age of forty-five, when you are wearing glasses or contacts, you will still have excellent distance vision, but you'll find you can't read well with them. In effect, the glasses and contacts simulate normal vision, so, just like a forty-five-year-old with farsightedness, reading becomes difficult.

At that point, you have a couple of options. You can wear reading glasses with your contacts. You can get bifocal lenses, which are glasses with a distance correction in the top half of the lens and a reading correction in the bottom half. The third option is to take off your glasses or contacts to read. Because you are nearsighted, you can see close up without glasses. Then put your glasses back on to see far away. This option works for some people but not others because their nearsightedness is often either too much or too little for optimal reading vision.

Presbyopia and Farsightedness

Farsightedness (hyperopia) is often confused with presbyopia because both impair near vision. Farsightedness impairs near vision because the natural focus of the eye falls behind the retina. Presbyopia impairs near vision because the lens becomes too stiff with age to focus up close. The combination of presbyopia and farsightedness is a double whammy to near vision as we age.

If you are young, hyperopia isn't too much of a problem. The focusing power of the natural lens when you are young can often overcome farsightedness, so you can see well both far and close. As the natural lens ages and hardens, it gradually loses its ability to compensate for the farsightedness. If you are hyperopic, you lose your reading vision earlier than other people, perhaps in your early forties. You get reading glasses. Then, as you get into your late forties or early fifties, you notice blurry distance vision, too, as the natural lens loses all ability to compensate for the farsightedness. At that point you get bifocals.

The exact ages vary from person to person but the pattern is nearly universal in hyperopic individuals: good overall vision in youth, followed by a gradual loss of near vision, and then later by a gradual blurring of distance vision. Glasses are often particularly frustrating for farsighted individuals because they never got used to them when they were young.

How Your Vision Is Measured

Part of an eye exam is measurement of *visual acuity.* Visual acuity is the clarity or sharpness of your vision. Normal visual acuity is described as 20/20 vision. That means that you can see at twenty feet what a person with normal vision can see at twenty feet. On the other hand, if your vision is 20/40, you can see at twenty feet what a person with normal vision can see at forty feet. Your vision is worse than normal. Visual acuity is determined by using the familiar eye chart with progressively smaller letters on each line. Some people can see 20/15 or 20/10, which is even better than 20/20. These people are said to have "super vision" or "supranormal vision." One of the great advances in LASIK over the last decade has been wavefront-guided LASIK. Wavefront is a greatly improved tool for analyzing the imperfections in the eye. It allows the eye surgeon to achieve better than 20/20 vision in most patients. Wavefront is discussed in more detail in chapter 5 on LASIK.

Numbers such as 20/20 or 20/40 describe your visual acuity but do not measure your refractive error—how inaccurately your eye bends, or refracts, light. When an eye doctor measures your refractive error, what you end up with is your eyeglass prescription.

Understanding Your Eyeglass Prescription

Most people correct their refractive error by wearing eyeglasses. Your eyeglass prescription is written in numbers. The type and degree of refractive error is quantified in units of measure called *diopters*. If you have ever wondered what those numbers mean, here is how to read and understand your prescription.

To arrive at your prescription, your doctor takes three measurements during the eye exam: sphere, cylinder, and axis. Your prescription for glasses may look something like this:

OD	– 1.25	sph			Add +2.00
OS	– 1.25	– 0.50	X	15	Add +2.00

OD and OS refer to the right and left eyes, respectively. The first row is the prescription for the right eye, and the second row is the prescription for the left eye. The first number in each row, next to OD or OS, represents the *sphere*. The sphere measure reveals whether you are nearsighted or farsighted. A negative diopter value indicates myopia, or nearsightedness. A positive diopter indicates hyperopia, or farsightedness. The higher the number, the worse the nearsightedness or farsightedness. In the example above, the person has mild myopia (–1.25 diopters) in both eyes.

The number in the second column represents the astigmatism. This number is also called *cylinder*. If the second column is not blank, you have some degree of astigmatism. The larger the number, the more astigmatism you have. In the example above, this person has –0.50 diopters of astigmatism in the left eye. In the right eye, there is no astigmatism, indicated by "sph," which is an abbreviation for "spherical."

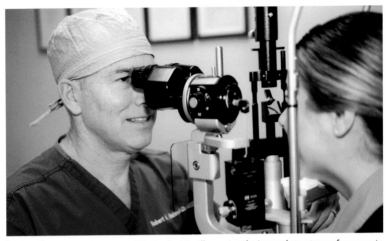

As part of your eye exam, your ophthalmologist will examine the internal structures of your eye to ensure that you don't have cataracts, macular degeneration, or other diseases.

If astigmatism is present, your eye doctor takes an *axis measurement.* The axis is the third column in the prescription. Recall that the eye is oval-shaped if you have astigmatism. The axis measurement indicates the angle of the oval shape relative to horizontal. In the prescription on the previous page, the astigmatism in the left eye is positioned at an angle of 15 degrees above the horizontal.

In some prescriptions, there is fourth column with the word *Add* followed by a number. This indicates a prescription for bifocal or progressive lenses. A "reading add" is a lens in the lower half of the glasses that provides additional help with reading when the wearer looks down. Reading adds are used in patients with presbyopia over the age of forty-five. In the prescription on the previous page, there is an extra boost of 2.00 diopters in the lower half of the glasses to allow this individual to read clearly.

In general, nearsightedness of 0 to −3.00 diopters is considered *mild,* −3.00 to −7.00 diopters is considered *moderate,* and −7.00 or more is *highly myopic.* For farsightedness, 0 to +1.50 is considered *mild,* +1.50 to +3.00 is considered *moderate,* and more than +3.00 is *highly hyperopic.* For astigmatism, less than 1.50 diopters is *mild,* 1.50 to 3.00 diopters is *moderate,* and more than 3.00 is *high astigmatism.*

2

Vision Correction Surgery: An Overview

If you've read this far, you know how the eye works. You know that you have a refractive error, which is a medical way of saying that you need glasses or contacts. You may have nearsightedness, farsightedness, or astigmatism, and, if you are over forty-five, you also likely have presbyopia impairing your reading vision. This chapter provides an overview of the various surgical procedures we use to correct your vision. The colloquial term for these procedures is *vision correction surgery*. Because these procedures correct refractive errors, eye doctors call these procedures *refractive surgery*. In this book we'll use both terms.

We can correct refractive errors by changing either the curvature of the cornea or the power of the lens of the eye. So refractive surgery divides neatly into two categories: *cornea-based refractive surgery* and *lens-based refractive surgery*.

Cornea-Based Refractive Surgery

There are two major corneal refractive surgeries: LASIK and PRK. Both are laser-based, very similar in method, and have the same long-term results, although PRK has a longer recovery.

Nearly everyone knows someone who has had a successful LASIK procedure. Most people come into our office asking for LASIK. Some are better candidates for a different procedure. An important part of our role is to educate them about their other options. There are some surgeons who pride themselves on being LASIK surgeons. We believe that it is important to be a complete refractive surgeon, not just a LASIK surgeon. We believe that a surgeon should master all of the procedures in *Figure 9* to properly take care of the range of patients we

The Spectrum of Refractive Surgery

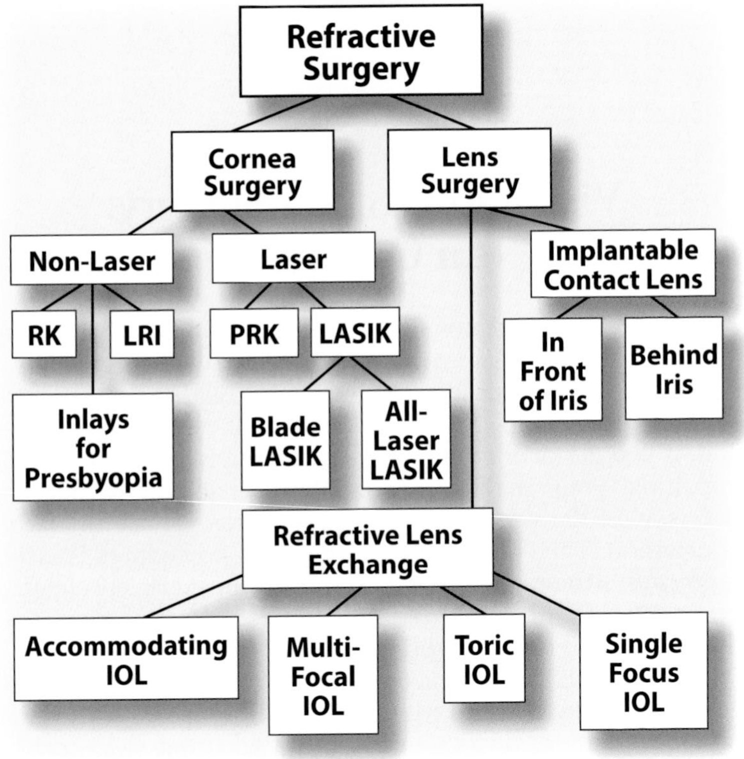

Figure 9. No one procedure is right for everyone. The surgeon needs to evaluate each patient individually and select the appropriate procedure.

see. There is an old saying that, if your only tool is a hammer, everything looks like a nail. This is the trap that surgeons who do only LASIK can fall into.

There are also non-laser cornea-based refractive surgeries, such as the new corneal inlays, which we will discuss later in this chapter.

LASIK

LASIK *(laser in-situ keratomileusis)* is the mainstay of refractive surgery today and is usually an excellent choice for low to moderate degrees of nearsightedness, farsightedness, and astigmatism. In LASIK, the surgeon makes a flap on the

The LASIK Procedure

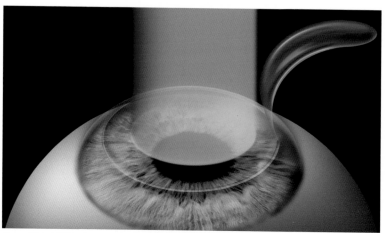

Figure 10. In LASIK, a laser separates the outer layers of the cornea, which are pulled back to make a flap. An excimer laser then reshapes the exposed surface to correct vision. The flap is replaced and sticks without sutures, allowing rapid healing.

surface of the cornea. The flap includes the outer layers of the cornea—the *epithelium* and part of the *stroma*. The flap is about as thick as a soft contact lens and attached at the upper part of the cornea, under the eyelid. The flap is folded back, exposing the underlying tissue (the stroma). An *excimer laser* is then applied in a preprogrammed, computer-controlled pattern to reshape the cornea *(Figure 10)*. The flap is replaced and sticks by itself, almost like Velcro. Replacing the flap restores all the layers of the cornea, so the healing is very fast.

The excimer laser is uniquely suited to the task of refractive surgery because it *ablates,* or vaporizes, tissue by breaking apart the molecules without heating the tissue left behind. The unparalleled precision of the excimer laser makes it the ultimate reshaping tool. Each pulse of the excimer laser removes only 1/100,000 inch of tissue. The laser is so precise that it would take 600 pulses to shave through one strand of human hair. This precision allows the surgeon to sculpt the cornea into the correct shape to allow rays of light to focus properly on the retina. The result is sharp vision without glasses or contacts.

There are two ways to make the flap. Traditionally, the flap was made with a fancy vibrating blade called a *microkeratome.*

This is usually called *blade LASIK*. Nowadays, the best way to make the flap is by using a *femtosecond laser*. This laser outlines the flap by creating a sheet of millions of tiny bubbles that separate the flap from the cornea. The femtosecond laser is very expensive, so there are still many surgeons using the older microkeratomes, but the trend is strongly toward laser flaps. A laser flap is more precise and safer than a microkeratome-created flap.

LASIK performed with a laser flap is called *all-laser LASIK*. All-laser LASIK takes about five minutes per eye and is a painless, in-office procedure. Recovery takes four to six hours. Most people see 20/20 or better the next day. LASIK is discussed in detail in a chapter 5.

PRK: LASIK without a Flap

PRK is an abbreviation for *photorefractive keratectomy*. PRK was the first refractive procedure done with a laser, and is the predecessor of LASIK. In PRK, the outer cell layer of the eye (the epithelium) is gently scraped away. This exposes the underlying stroma, a firm fibrous tissue that makes up the bulk of the cornea. The same excimer laser used in LASIK is then used to reshape the cornea, in exactly the same manner as in LASIK *(Figure 11)*. The PRK procedure takes about five minutes per eye and is painless.

Just as with LASIK, PRK can correct nearsightedness, farsightedness, and astigmatism. The main difference between PRK and LASIK is the speed of recovery. With LASIK, the healing is a matter of hours, and your vision is excellent the next day. With PRK, the outer cell layer, the epithelium, needs to regenerate. The epithelium takes about four days to completely recover the area of laser treatment. During these four days, your eye will be irritated and feel scratchy. It takes several weeks for the epithelium to become completely smooth. During these weeks your vision will be improved but not yet perfect.

There are several situations in which PRK is preferable to LASIK, despite the slower recovery. If you have a thinner-than-average cornea, there may not be enough tissue left after the LASIK flap is made to safely reshape the cornea with the laser. PRK is also preferable to LASIK if you are suspected of having a distortion in the cornea called *keratoconus*. You'll find more detailed information on PRK in chapter 6.

The PRK Procedure

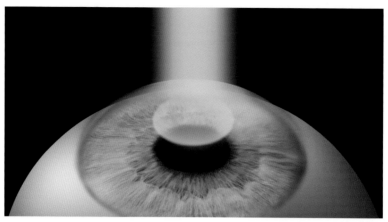

Figure 11. PRK is performed by directly shaping the outer layers of the cornea with an excimer laser. Unlike with LASIK, there is no flap.

Cornea-based refractive surgeries, such as LASIK and PRK, are appropriate for most people, but don't work as well for people with high degrees of myopia or hyperopia. For these individuals, lens-based refractive surgery is often preferable.

Lens-Based Refractive Surgery

Lens-based surgery involves inserting a new lens in the eye. The new lens has improved focusing power that can correct nearsightedness, farsightedness, and even astigmatism. The range of corrections possible with lens-based refractive surgery is far greater than with corneal surgery, and patients with very high degrees of myopia and hyperopia can be treated with excellent results and good image quality. There are two primary lens-based procedures: the implantable contact lens and refractive lens exchange.

The Implantable Contact Lens

Although LASIK is an excellent way to correct vision in most people with low and moderate levels of myopia, it is often not the best choice for high levels of myopia. When LASIK is used for high levels of myopia, patients can find that the clarity and quality of vision, particularly at night, is not as good as with glasses or contacts. For these patients we prefer the implantable contact lens, or ICL.

Implantable Contact Lens

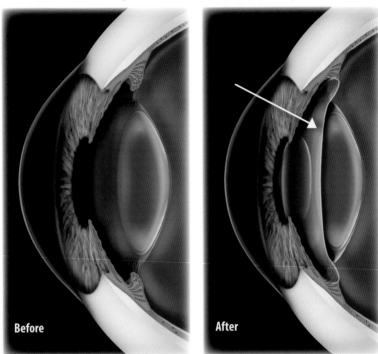

Figure 12. The arrow shows the implantable contact lens (ICL), which has been inserted behind the iris (the colored part of the eye), in front of the natural lens. An ICL can correct high levels of nearsightedness.

The implantable contact lens is a tiny, soft lens, about a quarter of an inch in diameter, that is inserted behind the iris, in front of the natural lens *(Figure 12)*. To do this, the surgeon makes a small incision, about three millimeters wide, at the junction of the cornea and sclera. The lens is rolled up, inserted through the incision, and then unrolled in the eye. The lens is then tucked in position behind the iris. The procedure is painless, takes about seven minutes per eye, and is done under twilight anesthesia. You can see better immediately afterward, usually well enough to read a clock on a wall across the room. Most people see 20/20 or better the next day.

I generally recommend the ICL to patients whose myopia is worse than −8.00 diopters. I also sometimes recommend it to people whose myopia is less than −8.00 diopters, but who have some contraindication to LASIK and PRK. Currently, the ICL is not available for hyperopia. The implantable contact lens is discussed in detail in chapter 7.

Refractive Lens Exchange

If you have hyperopia, or farsightedness, refractive lens exchange may be your best option. Refractive lens exchange, or *RLE* for short, involves removing your natural lens and replacing it with a synthetic lens. The surgeon makes a small incision at the junction of the cornea and sclera and inserts a tiny vibrating probe. The probe is used to break up the natural lens into tiny pieces and vacuum it out. A new synthetic lens is rolled up and inserted into the eye. It is unrolled in the eye in the space that the natural lens formerly occupied *(Figure 13)*.

The procedure is painless, takes about ten minutes per eye, and is performed while you are under twilight anesthesia. The recovery is also painless and patients typically have excellent vision the next day.

RLE is the same operation as cataract surgery, but is done for patients who don't have a cataract. More than 3 million cataract surgeries are done in the United States each year. Because of this high volume, cataract surgery has become highly advanced and very safe. RLE benefits from these advances and experience. In particular, over the past few decades, highly advanced synthetic lenses have become available. Some of these lenses correct astigmatism, while others are designed to correct presbyopia by restoring both reading and distance vision. These lenses are discussed in the following chapters.

Because LASIK can also correct farsightedness, the choice between LASIK and RLE can be a subtle one. We generally lean toward RLE for higher corrections because the effect of LASIK for high hyperopic corrections can wear off over time. We also recommend RLE if your vision problem is particularly amenable to solution with one of the advanced synthetic lenses, such as the bifocal or astigmatism correcting lenses. If you have the beginnings of a cataract, we much prefer RLE, recognizing that we can fix the vision and cure the early cataract with a single procedure.

Refractive Lens Exchange

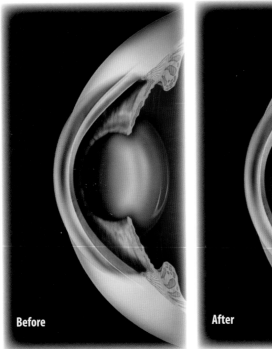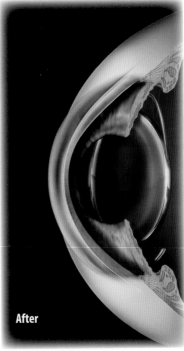

Before   **After**

Figure 13. In a refractive lens exchange (RLE), the natural lens is removed and replaced with a synthetic lens. The surgeon chooses a lens with the power to provide clearly focused vision.

Other Refractive Procedures

LASIK, PRK, the implantable contact lens, and refractive lens exchange are the appropriate procedures for almost everyone. There are a variety of other procedures, some of which are obsolete and some of which are still relevant, but they are less commonly done. The full spectrum of refractive surgery is shown in Figure 9 on page 16.

In addition to laser corneal surgeries, there are also incisional corneal surgeries. *Radial keratotomy,* the old Russian procedure, is one example, but is obsolete now. *Limbal relaxing incisions* are a cousin procedure that is very much used today. One or two small incisions are made at the edge of the cornea *(Figure 14).* Limbal relaxing incisions are a good way

Limbal Relaxing Incisions

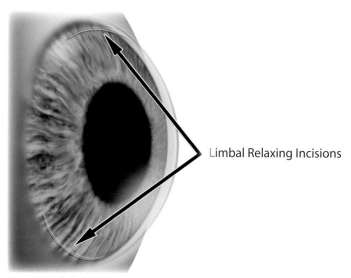

Limbal Relaxing Incisions

Figure 14. Limbal relaxing incisions are small incisions made at the outer edge of the cornea. These incisions cause the oval cornea to relax, transforming it into a round shape; this change in shape corrects astigmatism.

to correct low to moderate amounts of astigmatism in combination with RLE or an ICL.

Another non-laser option, the *corneal inlay,* is a tiny clear lens that is inserted into a pocket created in the center of the cornea. The inlay acts like a reading lens and is designed to correct presbyopia. Because of slow healing and variable results, we generally don't recommend these corneal inlays. This is a new procedure and research is continuing.

Getting Rid of Reading Glasses

LASIK and the other surgeries described in this chapter allow us to set the focus of your eyes for excellent distance vision, excellent near vision, or anywhere in between. If you are under forty-five years old, we normally set the focus of your eyes for excellent distance vision. Because the natural lenses in your eyes are still flexible, you will also have good intermediate and near vision after surgery.

If you are over forty-five, presbyopia is setting in. It is easy to give you excellent distance vision with LASIK and the other surgeries discussed previously. The challenge is giving you good near and intermediate vision, too. There are several approaches we use to meet this challenge, which we'll review in this section.

Monovision

The most common solution to presbyopia is *monovision.* In monovision, we correct one eye for excellent distance vision, and we set the focus of your other eye for close vision.

To be more precise, the close eye can be set for either intermediate or near vision. If you spend a lot of time on a computer, we set the close eye for intermediate vision. If a computer is not a major part of your life, we often set the close eye for near vision, so you can read a menu in a dimly lit restaurant. Each of the procedures discussed previously can be used to create a monovision correction.

Monovision sounds strange, but for many people it works very well. People with successful monovision see both far and close effortlessly; they can drive a car and read a menu in a restaurant without glasses. In many people, the brain is wired to automatically select the eye with better vision, so you aren't even aware of which eye you are using to see at any moment. Monovision is similar to stereo sound, where each ear hears something slightly different, but the brain puts the information from the ears together into a single sound field.

Monovision is great, but not perfect. With monovision, distance vision is not quite as sharp as having both eyes corrected for distance, but it is about 90 to 95 percent as sharp. You may notice the lack of perfect sharpness particularly at night, while driving, because there is less light. In that case we can prescribe a pair of glasses for night driving that correct your near eye for distance vision, but this is usually not necessary.

Some people don't tolerate monovision well. Perhaps they don't like the slight sacrifice in clarity of distance vision. Others find that the brain doesn't switch between eyes naturally or that having different vision in the eyes doesn't work well for them.

The key to successful monovision is testing you before surgery to see if you will like it. This testing can be done in the office with temporary glasses. With these glasses you can experience monovision before you have surgery. Monovision testing can also be done with temporary contact lenses. We place these contacts in your eyes in the office. You wear them for a few days, even while sleeping, and then we remove them. This allows you to experience monovision in the real world, outside the office. You see what it is like to drive, work on a computer, and read your cell phone or newspaper.

Monovision correction can be achieved with LASIK, implantable contact lenses, or refractive lens exchange. Which procedure is the best way to achieve a monovision correction depends on the patient. Generally, for lower levels of correction we do monovision with LASIK. For higher levels of farsightedness we often use refractive lens exchange, and for higher levels of nearsightedness we often use implantable lenses.

Monovision is a great solution for presbyopia for many people, but it is not for everyone. The other approach to treating presbyopia is refractive lens exchange with advanced lens implants.

Multifocal Lens Implants

With refractive lens exchange (RLE), we remove the natural lens and replace it with an improved synthetic lens that provides a better focus for your eyes. One of the benefits of RLE is the ability to use *multifocal lens implants*. These are implants that can correct presbyopia.

Most lens implants have a single focal point, for either far or intermediate or near vision. These are called single-focus or *monofocal lenses*. You get clear vision at one of these three distances, but only one. Multifocal implants *(Figure 15)* are designed to give you clear vision for both far and near. A series of concentric rings on the lens bends light to create two focal points. With a multifocal lens you can watch television and read a menu without glasses.

For some people, multifocal lenses are a great option. However, there are two compromises with these lenses. The first is that distance vision is not quite as sharp as with a monofocal lens because only half of the incoming light is focused perfectly for distance (the other half is focused for reading). This can create an annoying blur that feels like

Multifocal Lens Implant

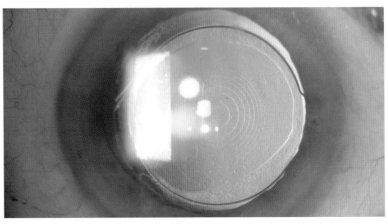

Figure 15. A multifocal lens, shown here inside the eye after surgery, has a series of concentric rings that allow for both far and close vision without glasses. Once inserted, the implanted lenses are not visible to others.

wearing dirty glasses. The second compromise is that the rings on the lens that create the multifocal effect cause rings around headlights and streetlights at night.

You may find that you are somewhat confused about what is the best vision correction option for you. Don't feel bad. It takes the average eye doctor the first six months of training to understand the various procedures described above. If you are over forty-five years old, and likely have presbyopia, we would suggest that you read this chapter twice. Then ask your eye surgeon to explain how the general information presented here applies to you. The bottom line is this: you should go into your vision correction procedure understanding what can be done to optimize your close vision after surgery and for the rest of your life.

3

Are You a Candidate for Vision Correction Surgery?

When you are considering vision correction surgery, it's important to become an informed consumer. You want to know about the various surgical options available, as well as whether you are a good candidate for surgery. Can everyone have surgery and get rid of their glasses? The answer is: it depends on a variety of physical, occupational, and motivational factors. In this chapter, we'll explain the factors involved in determining whether you're a good candidate for vision correction surgery.

Physical Factors

To be considered a good candidate for vision correction surgery, it's important to be in overall good health. We eye doctors check for specific factors that could affect the outcome of your eye surgery.

Ideal Age

A good candidate is at least eighteen years old because the vision of people younger than eighteen years usually continues to change. Myopia may continue to increase in some patients until their mid to late twenties. Surgery can be done, but the vision after surgery will gradually decline, just as it was declining before surgery.

As with all rules, there are exceptions. We once consulted with a sixteen-year-old who was the star of his high school football team. He could no longer tolerate the discomfort of his contacts and couldn't play effectively with glasses. He underwent LASIK with excellent results, but understood that he'd be back in five or ten years for an enhancement procedure to better his vision as age-related changes occurred.

Stable Prescription

No matter what your age, to be considered a good candidate for vision correction surgery, your eyeglass prescription for distance should be stable. In practical terms, your prescription is stable if your glasses or contacts are at least a year old and you still see well with them. Reading glasses are a different story. You may need stronger reading glasses every few years as the lens of your eye hardens, but this is not a sign of instability of your prescription.

Treatable Refractive Parameters

The optimal procedure will depend on your eyeglass prescription. Refer back to the opening chapter for an explanation of how to read your eyeglass prescription. Very generally, myopia up to −8.00 diopters and hyperopia up to +3.00 diopters is treated with either PRK or LASIK. Farsightedness more than +3.00 diopters is usually treated with refractive lens exchange. Myopia above −8.00 diopters is best treated with a contact lens implant.

Eye Health

Your eyes should be healthy. You shouldn't have serious eye diseases or prior major eye surgeries or injuries. Your cornea should be structurally normal, not irregularly shaped (this will be determined at your preoperative examination). In particular, it is best if both eyes can be corrected to 20/20 vision with glasses.

Pupil Size

One of the side effects of vision correction surgery is an increase in halos and starburst. These night-vision disturbances occur when you are in a dark environment and look at a small bright light, such as a headlight or a streetlight. Halo is the glow that surrounds the light source, and starburst refers to the little spiky rays of light that emanate from the light source. If you have unusually large pupils, more light enters your eyes at night. Some doctors believe that this extra light causes more starburst and halos. A number of major studies have now shown that this is not the case—there is no correlation between pupil size and night vision. We believe, and more and more doctors are coming to agree, that pupil size is unimportant to your candidacy for vision correction surgery.

Medical Conditions

The following conditions represent areas of controversy in terms of whether a patient is a good candidate for vision correction surgery. Our approach is to evaluate these conditions on a case-by-case basis. If you have any of these conditions, discuss them with your eye surgeon.

Pregnancy

Most eye surgeons consider pregnancy a contraindication to surgery. It isn't that surgery, or the medicines involved, have been shown to have any risk to the fetus. Rather, we worry that if a baby is born with a birth defect, the mother might blame herself, and us, for the birth defect. Also, vision can sometimes change late in pregnancy, which could make the results of vision correction surgery less accurate. In certain situations we will do LASIK in the first or second trimester, but we don't give the usual eyedrops and oral sedative to be sure not to expose the fetus to any medications.

Breastfeeding

Some doctors are concerned that vision may change while a mother is nursing. This is not our experience. If more than two months have passed since delivery, you are a candidate for vision correction surgery. However, if you are nursing and do have the surgery, we recommend you avoid oral sedatives, such as Valium, because the drugs will affect your breast milk.

Autoimmune Diseases

Autoimmune diseases are ailments caused by an abnormal attack by your immune system on the natural, healthy cells of your body. These diseases include lupus, Hashimoto's thyroiditis, and rheumatoid arthritis. Certain autoimmune diseases, such as rheumatoid arthritis, have been associated with melting of the cornea or sclera in patients who have eye surgery, although only rarely. These conditions can also cause severe dry eye. In general, if you have a well-controlled autoimmune disease, are under age sixty-five, and don't have significant dryness in your eyes, you are still often a good candidate for vision correction surgery.

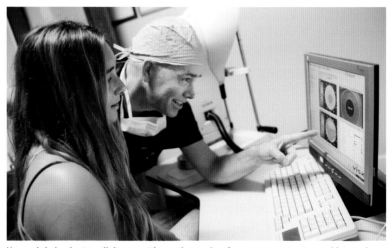

Your ophthalmologist will discuss with you the results of your eye examination and let you know what your options are for corrective surgery.

Diabetic Retinopathy

Diabetic retinopathy is a potentially blinding complication of diabetes that can damage the retina. Patients with diabetes who do not have retinal disease are usually candidates for LASIK or PRK, but may not be for lens-based surgeries.

Prescription Medications

Certain prescription medicines may sometimes affect the results of surgery. Accutane, used to treat severe acne, can make the eyes drier after surgery. *Oral corticosteroids,* like prednisone, are sometimes used by individuals with severe allergies, asthma, or autoimmune diseases such as arthritis and lupus. These drugs can increase eye pressure and increase your chance of getting a cataract. Tell your eye doctor about any prescription and over-the-counter medications you are taking.

Occupational Factors

Certain occupations may make you a poorer candidate for vision correction surgery. Starburst at night after surgery is a minor hindrance to most people, but if you are a truck driver whose living depends on driving extensively at night, night-vision disturbances could be a major problem. LASIK can be a positive or a negative for professional athletes. In Los Angeles, where we practice ophthalmology, we try to avoid performing

LASIK on the LA Dodgers' baseball players because they need to be able to spot a fly ball descending at speed under the stadium lights. On the other hand, for other professional athletes whose contact lenses are an uncomfortable distraction during games, LASIK can raise their performance a notch.

Vision correction surgery can be lifesaving for those who put their lives in harm's way: our police, firefighters, and military personnel. After surgery, these individuals never have to worry about losing their glasses or contacts in a moment of crisis. All the U.S. military services now permit vision correction surgery. Most police and fire departments require a minimal level of vision without glasses. LASIK can help you meet these requirements and open up a career that would otherwise be closed to you. Many police, fire, and military services require a waiting period after surgery before you can go on active duty. Make sure you understand service requirements before having the surgery.

Patient Expectations

We surgeons try hard to give everyone perfect vision after surgery. We nearly always achieve very good vision, but we don't always get all the way to perfect. Some individuals come into our office unhappy with their vision with their glasses and contacts. They don't mind wearing the glasses or contacts, but they simply are not seeing well enough, even with glasses on or contacts in. These patients may be disappointed after surgery because the procedure often leaves their vision the same as with their glasses or contacts.

The ideal motivation for surgery is that you dislike your glasses and contacts and would be happy if your vision after surgery were very good, even if it weren't quite perfect. If that's your expectation, you will almost surely be happy after vision correction surgery.

4

The Preoperative Evaluation

At most eye surgery centers, including our center, the preoperative evaluation occurs in two steps. Step one is the initial consultation, and step two is a comprehensive eye exam.

Initial Consultation

The purpose of the initial consultation with an eye surgeon is to help you decide whether to have surgery and which procedure you want to have. Your preoperative evaluation is your chance to figure this out by consulting with an expert surgeon. This consultation takes about an hour to an hour and a half, and is often complimentary. During the initial consultation, some basic measurements are taken of your eyes.

You should do four things to prepare for your initial consultation. First, make a list of the questions you want answered. A written list ensures that you don't forget anything and helps the surgery center be sure you are fully informed. Second, bring all the glasses you routinely wear, and your contact lens prescription if you have it handy.

The third preparatory step is to stop wearing your contact lenses for seventy-two hours prior to the appointment (other centers may request a longer or shorter period). Just as shoes can distort the shape of your toes, contacts can distort the shape of your cornea. After seventy-two hours, most people's corneas return to their normal shapes. A normal corneal shape is important for the surgeon in taking accurate measurements.

The fourth preparatory step is to gather your medical and eye history information. Get together a list of your medical problems and current medications, including over-the-counter meds. If you have had previous eye surgery, know the dates and the procedures that were done. Old records can be helpful, if available. If your vision has changed recently, old prescriptions are useful so the surgeon can see how much change has occurred.

Your preoperative consultation shouldn't be rushed. You shouldn't feel like you are on an assembly line. You should have the opportunity to ask as many questions as necessary in order to feel safe and comfortable undergoing surgery. You may want to invite a friend, your spouse, or another family member to sit in on the meeting with the surgeon. He or she may help you remember questions to ask or may help you recall information later.

You shouldn't feel pressured to have surgery. Unfortunately, some LASIK centers use a high-pressure sales approach, almost like selling used cars. There is some chance that these centers may recommend surgery even if you are not a good candidate. If you feel you are getting a sales push, leave. LASIK is a surgical procedure and should be treated as such.

If you want to proceed with surgery, the next step is the comprehensive eye exam. This may be done at the same appointment as the consultation, or you may return at a later date for this part of the preoperative evaluation. A careful eye exam is necessary to be sure your eyes are healthy and to find any conditions that might result in a less-than-optimal result. In the preceding chapter, we indicated some of the most common conditions, but those were only a small fraction of the possible conditions that affect the eyes. The surgeon's responsibility is to make sure there aren't any others, and, if there are, to let you know about them and discuss them with you.

Comprehensive Eye Examination

The comprehensive eye examination will determine if you are a good candidate for the recommended procedure by uncovering any eye conditions that may impair your outcome. Also, your eyes will be carefully measured to achieve the optimal result from the chosen procedure.

Your comprehensive exam will likely take an hour to an hour and a half. A variety of tests and exams will be done. Following is a brief overview. Whoever is doing the tests

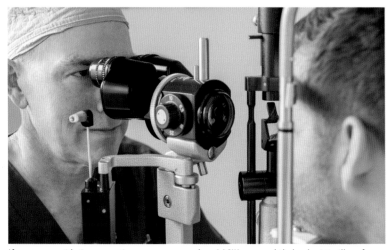

If you are considering corrective eye surgery, such as LASIK, your ophthalmologist will perform a more in-depth exam of your eye structures to determine whether you are a good candidate for surgery.

should explain them to you as they are done. None of these tests are painful.

Visual Acuity Test

Visual acuity refers to the clarity of your vision. (*Acuity* is from the Latin *acuitas,* which means "sharpness.") In other words, how well do you see? Your eye doctor will use the familiar eye chart most of us know, called the *Snellen chart.* It was named after the nineteenth-century Dutch ophthalmologist Hermann Snellen, who invented it. It consists of rows of black letters—very large at the top, very small at the bottom—against a white background. Each eye will be tested separately while the other eye is covered.

The result of your visual acuity test is expressed by a phrase such as "20/20 vision" or "20/40 vision," which some people find confusing. The first number, in the United States at least, is always 20—which is the distance, in feet, you're sitting from the eye chart. (Where the metric system is used, the first number is 6, indicating that the patient is sitting 6 meters from the chart.)

The second number conveys how much your visual acuity differs from normal eyesight. If you have 20/20 vision, you can see at twenty feet what other people with normal vision can see at twenty feet. If your vision is 20/40, you can see at twenty feet what people with normal vision can see at forty feet. The higher the second number, the worse your vision. At 20/200 vision or worse, we consider you *legally blind* without glasses. If your vision is this bad, you are completely disabled if you lose your glasses or contacts.

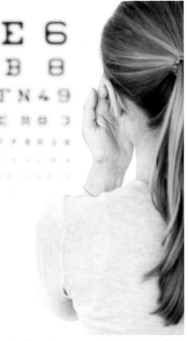

Intraocular Pressure Measurement

We measure the pressure in your eye to look for glaucoma. Glaucoma is a condition of elevated eye pressure that gradually damages the optic nerve. The eye is numbed with drops and a device called a *tonometer* touches the eye and measures the pressure inside.

The Snellen chart measures the clarity of your vision at a distance of twenty feet.

Testing for Dry Eyes

One of the side effects of LASIK and PRK is that your eyes can feel drier. The amount of tears you produce and the quality of tears will be evaluated in several ways. If your eyes are adequately moist before surgery, significant dryness is usually not an issue afterward.

Anterior Segment Examination

The doctor will examine the front part of your eye, called the *anterior segment,* which includes the eyelids, cornea, iris, and lens. Using a powerful biomicroscope, she will check for infection, inflammation of the eyelids, diseases of the cornea, and signs of cataract. Any of these conditions may disqualify you as a good candidate for vision correction surgery.

Examination of the Retina and Optic Nerve

The doctor will inspect the retina, blood vessels, and optic nerve at the back of the eye for signs of macular degeneration or nerve damage. This part of the exam is traditionally done by dilating the eyes and looking through a device called an *ophthalmoscope*. People don't like having their eyes dilated because their vision remains blurry for hours. For most patients in our center, we are able to use a retinal camera to take a photo of the retina and nerve, avoiding the need to dilate the eyes. This technology is becoming more widely available.

Informed Consent

If your doctor determines that you are a candidate for vision correction surgery, he or she will ask you to sign an informed consent form. This is your written, legal consent to have the surgeon proceed with your vision correction surgery. Review this form carefully. It should not read like a legal document, but should explain clearly and simply the risks and benefits of the surgery. Sign it only after you understand everything on the form. Don't be shy about asking questions. Signing the consent form doesn't obligate you to have the surgery—you can always change your mind later.

5

LASIK

For most people, LASIK is the best way to permanently correct their vision. However, LASIK isn't the right procedure for everyone. In this chapter, we'll discuss who is a good candidate and who isn't. We'll talk about the preparation for and the recovery from LASIK. We'll also review the results you can expect and discuss possible problems and complications.

How LASIK Corrects Your Vision

As discussed in chapter 2, a LASIK procedure involves using a laser to reshape the cornea so that it changes the way light travels through the cornea and onto the retina. During the LASIK procedure, the outermost layers of the cornea are separated, creating a thin flap, which is gently folded back, exposing the stromal tissue beneath. The exposed corneal tissue is then precisely sculpted by an excimer laser into a new shape to correct your vision. The flap is set back in place and is held in position by the cornea's natural stickiness, almost like Velcro. Doing LASIK on your eyes is analogous to sculpting a contact lens onto the surface of your eye—you see clearly, but without the routine of removing, cleaning, or changing a contact lens.

LASIK and Myopic Correction

As explained earlier, an individual who is nearsighted (myopic) has a cornea with too much curvature in proportion to the length of their eye. Once the corneal flap is made and lifted back, the excimer laser reshapes the underlying stroma by removing more tissue from the center of the cornea than from the periphery. The result is a flatter cornea with less

LASIK Reshapes the Cornea

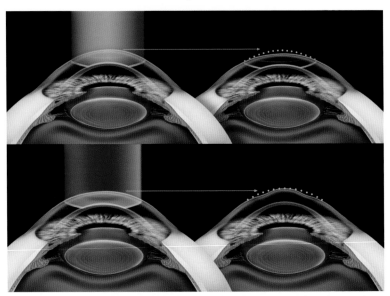

Figure 16. Top: To correct nearsightedness, the excimer laser removes tissue from the central part of the cornea. This reduces the curvature of the cornea and causes the incoming light to focus correctly. *Bottom:* To correct farsightedness, the laser does the opposite: it removes tissue from the periphery of the cornea, increasing its curvature.

focusing power. The surgeon's careful, precise measurements are programmed into the computer to guide the excimer laser. When the reshaping is complete, the flap is replaced *(Figure 16. Top)*. The result is that light rays coming through the cornea now come to a point of focus on the retina rather than in front of it.

LASIK and Hyperopic Correction

A farsighted (hyperopic) patient, on the other hand, has a cornea that is not curved enough for the length of their eye. The excimer laser is programmed to remove tissue predominantly from the periphery of the cornea, leaving the center of the cornea untouched; this creates more of a domed shape *(Figure 16. Bottom)* The increased curvature of the cornea allows light rays to focus on the retina rather than behind it.

LASIK and Astigmatism

To treat astigmatism, the excimer laser removes tissue in an oval shape, correcting the shape of the cornea in one direction more than the other. The goal is to eliminate the oval shape of the corneal surface so that light rays passing through the cornea meet at a single point of focus on the retina. Astigmatism can be corrected with the laser in combination with correcting nearsightedness or farsightedness.

LASIK and Presbyopia

LASIK can treat presbyopia by creating a monovision correction. We can use LASIK to correct one eye for excellent distance vision and the other eye for excellent reading vision.

Are You a Candidate for LASIK?

The best candidates for LASIK have an eyeglass prescription that isn't extreme. If you are nearsighted, this means you may have myopia of up to –8.00 diopters. If you are farsighted, your hyperopia may be up to +3.00 diopters. Your level of astigmatism may be as high as +4.00 diopters. Patients outside of these ranges can still have LASIK, but they require a greater degree of corneal reshaping and expectations for crisp, clear vision are lower. Above –8.00 diopters of myopia, we usually recommend the implantable contact lens. Above +3.00 diopters of hyperopia, we prefer refractive lens exchange. Both of these options are covered in detail in later chapters.

Factors that May Prevent You from Having LASIK

The following conditions may make you a poor candidate, or at least a less-than-ideal candidate, for LASIK. Although the conditions listed are generally contraindications to LASIK, many are not absolute contraindications. If you have one of these conditions, consultation with an experienced LASIK surgeon will help you determine whether LASIK is still a possibility for you.

Thin Cornea

LASIK will not weaken a normal cornea, but if your cornea is unusually thin, LASIK could weaken it, causing distortion in your vision. If you have a thin cornea, PRK may be a better option for you. PRK is covered in detail in chapter 6.

Keratoconus

Keratoconus is an uncommon, hereditary condition that weakens the cornea. The weak cornea bulges outward gradually over time, just as a bicycle tire with a weak spot develops a bulge. Patients with this condition suffer from increasing nearsightedness, astigmatism, and poor vision. Keratoconus progresses gradually in younger people and then stabilizes around the age of forty.

Unfortunately, the LASIK flap can make this condition worse, so LASIK is not an option for patients with keratoconus. Sometimes, patients with this condition can be treated with PRK instead. An essential part of your preoperative exam is examining you for keratoconus, using specialized diagnostic mapping of the cornea.

Cataract

A cataract is a clouding of the lens within the eye that causes blurry vision. If you have a cataract, LASIK can accentuate the blurring of vision caused by the cataract. Patients with a cataract are usually good candidates for refractive lens exchange because refractive lens exchange corrects both the vision and the cataract. RLE is covered in detail in chapter 8.

Basement Membrane Dystrophy

Basement membrane dystrophy is a hereditary condition that causes the epithelium, the clear skin that covers the cornea, to slough off spontaneously, creating a corneal abrasion. It is a relatively common condition. People with basement membrane dystrophy can develop corneal abrasions after LASIK. These can cause discomfort and a slow recovery of vision after the procedure.

Prior Episodes of Herpes Keratitis

The same herpes virus that causes cold sores on the lips can cause recurring infection in the eye, resulting in scarring and blurred vision. LASIK can cause a reactivation of the virus. LASIK can often be done safely by pretreatment with drugs that suppress the virus. Note: this herpes virus is different from the virus that causes genital herpes, which is a sexually transmitted disease.

Significant Dry Eye

LASIK makes the eyes somewhat drier, so patients who have very dry eyes to start with can be somewhat uncomfortable after LASIK. Mild dry eye can also make wearing contact lenses very uncomfortable. All in all, people with mild dry eye often do much better with LASIK than with contact lenses. The surgeon will evaluate your tear production and advise you if LASIK is a good alternative for you. LASIK and dry eye are discussed in more detail later in this chapter.

The LASIK Flap

The eye surgeon starts the LASIK procedure by making a flap in the cornea. Many people become anxious when they hear this, because they don't like the idea of surgery in the delicate tissues of their outer eye. We can understand that feeling, but I want you to understand that this flap approach to surgery is a wonderful thing because it results in very rapid healing. The flap includes the epithelium, the outer layer of the cornea, and part of the underlying stroma, the middle, fibrous layer of the cornea. The epithelium is basically a clear skin over the eye. The epithelium has a huge number of nerves, more than any other part of your body. When the epithelium is injured, it hurts. Perhaps you've had a corneal abrasion from a contact lens or from trauma. If so, you know how painful an injury to the epithelium is.

When we make a flap on your eye, we lift the epithelium intact. When the flap is replaced at the end of the LASIK procedure, the epithelium is then replaced uninjured. This has great advantages: within a couple of hours your eyes are quite comfortable, and your vision is excellent in a few hours, too. And, as mentioned, using the flap approach means a very fast recovery.

There are two ways to make the flap. Traditionally, the flap was made with a specialized knife called a microkeratome. In concept, the microkeratome is similar to a deli meat slicer, with a vibrating cutting blade and a slot through which the flap emerges. The microkeratome is a reasonable way to make a LASIK flap, but it has two limitations. The first limitation is that the flap is not of uniform thickness. This may result in a less precise correction afterward. The second limitation is that occasionally the microkeratome can cut a hole through the flap. This complication requires terminating the LASIK procedure. The better way to make the flap is with all-laser LASIK.

All-Laser LASIK

All-laser LASIK creates the flap using a laser instead of a microkeratome. The laser used is not an excimer laser, but rather a different type of laser called a *femtosecond laser*. The femtosecond laser is scanned, under computer control, just below the surface of the cornea. The laser creates thousands of tiny bubbles that outline a perfect flap of a uniform thickness. The bubbles separate the flap from the cornea, allowing the flap to be created and lifted without using a knife or blade. This method is also called *blade-free LASIK*.

All-laser LASIK has two advantages over standard LASIK. First, with the all-laser approach, problems with the flap are very rare and easily handled. Second, the result of the laser treatment is more accurate. Studies by the U.S. Navy have shown a higher percentage of patients achieve 20/15 vision with all-laser LASIK compared to standard LASIK.

Seeing Better than 20/20 with LASIK

If you've had an eye exam, there was a part of the exam where the doctor asked you, "Which is better, one or two?" The doctor was using a device called a *phoropter* to measure your refractive error. He then gave you glasses or contact lenses to correct your refractive error so you could see 20/20. Usually, he didn't try to correct to better than 20/20. In fact, in decades past, most eye charts stopped at 20/20, so the doctor couldn't measure whether your vision was better than 20/20 even if he wanted to. Many doctors still feed these same phoropter measurements into their excimer lasers for LASIK, with the same result.

When we started doing LASIK procedures, in 1991, we thought that achieving 20/20 vision was a great result. After all, 20/20 is considered normal vision, and our patients who had been coping with poor vision for decades were delighted to have 20/20 vision. But while most normal people see 20/20, some people can see even better than that if the focusing power of their eye is optimized. People with 20/15 or better vision can see the spin on a tennis ball, or can see a golf ball on a green 200 yards away.

The famous test pilot Chuck Yeager, the first pilot to ever fly faster than the speed of sound, reportedly had 20/10 vision, which is twice as good as 20/20. This was part of the reason he was a fighter ace in World War II—because he could see enemy planes long before they could see him.

Many great baseball hitters, like Manny Ramirez, have vision of 20/15 or 20/10. This lets them see the ball sooner when it leaves the pitcher's hand. We say these people have "super vision" or "supranormal vision."

At the end of the 1990s, David Williams at the University of Rochester asked why more people didn't see better than 20/20. Studies found that everyone has imperfections in the way the eye focuses light, even after the myopia, hyperopia, or astigmatism are corrected by glasses or contacts. These imperfections are called *higher-order aberrations.* They prevent the average person from seeing better than 20/20. As mentioned earlier, a new technology called wavefront-guided LASIK now lets us achieve super vision in the majority of our patients.

Wavefront-Guided LASIK

A good way to think about higher-order aberrations is that each point on the eye has a slightly different refractive error. Put another way, each point on the eye needs a slightly different eyeglass prescription to correct it perfectly. When an eye doctor typically checks your eye for imperfections (refractive error), he or she measures only one point—the center of the pupil. Wavefront technology measures the eye at 1200 points, making the assessment of the eye much more precise.

Fortunately, a lot was known about higher-order aberrations even before they were discovered in the human eye. Astronomers have problems with higher-order aberrations from their telescope lenses and from the atmosphere itself. Astronomers had already developed a way to measure higher-order aberrations using a sophisticated device called a *wavefront analyzer.* They used these measurements to sharpen the image of distant galaxies.

Researchers applied wavefront analyzers to measure the higher-order aberrations of the human eye. Instead of measuring only one point on the eye, a wavefront analyzer measures 1,200 different points on the eye. This measurement provides a more detailed map of the eye's higher-order aberrations. These measurements are fed into the excimer laser, and the laser corrects not only the myopia, hyperopia, or astigmatism, but also the higher-order aberrations. The result is that many more people can see 20/15 or even better. With the data from the wavefront analysis, an ophthalmologist can now perform LASIK surgery that detects, measures, and corrects both low-order and higher-order aberrations. This process of measurement and treatment of higher-order aberrations is called *wavefront-guided LASIK (Figure 17)*.

Patients who undergo wavefront-guided LASIK have a faster recovery, sharper vision, and fewer side effects. A study at the Naval Medical Center in San Diego compared the results of Navy patients who had had conventional LASIK with the results of those who had had wavefront-guided LASIK. The results of the study indicated that 88 percent of conventional LASIK patients had achieved 20/20 or better vision six months after surgery. In contrast, 97 percent of the wavefront-guided LASIK patients had achieved 20/20 or better vision after the same time period.

Dr. Edward Manche and his research group at Stanford University compared wavefront-guided LASIK to conventional LASIK to determine which treatment was more effective in producing supranormal vision—vision better than 20/20. In the wavefront-guided group of eyes, 56 percent achieved vision of 20/12 or better. That is vision good enough for professional baseball. In contrast, only 41 percent of the eyes treated with conventional LASIK achieved 20/12 vision, although this is still a very respectable result.

Wavefront-guided LASIK may actually prevent some of the side effects that occur more often with conventional LASIK. Some patients who undergo conventional LASIK have problems with starburst or halos around lights at night or in dim lighting. These side effects usually occur because conventional LASIK can increase some higher-order aberrations. Because wavefront-guided LASIK is designed to correct these higher-order aberrations, such side effects are less likely to occur.

Wavefront-Guided LASIK

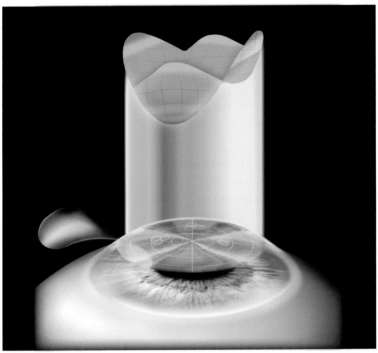

Figure 17. Wavefront technology allows an ophthalmologist to measure your eye's imperfections at 1,200 points on the eye, compared to only a single, central point measured by older technology, used for eyeglasses. With the use of wavefront, you can achieve better than 20/20 vision.

The Naval study showed that 30 percent of conventional LASIK patients reported an increase in seeing halos around lights at night, especially when driving. None of the wavefront-guided LASIK patients reported this side effect. Overall, the study concluded that wavefront-guided LASIK offers patients better quality of vision than conventional LASIK, and it significantly decreases night-vision problems, such as halos or starburst. Wavefront patients reported a greater level of satisfaction with their results than the conventional LASIK group did.

In practical terms, getting better than 20/20 vision isn't that important; most people are very happy with 20/20 after having had poor vision for much of their life. But super-clear vision is very nice, indeed. You can go to a baseball game and see the expression on the pitcher's face or read a street sign from a quarter mile away. You can sit in the back row of a movie theater and see every detail on the screen.

Sight is precious. We believe that your eyes should have the best possible treatment. It should be clear that wavefront-guided, all-laser LASIK is the best way to perform LASIK. It is what we use for all our LASIK patients to get the best possible distance vision. The U.S. Navy agrees with us: all jet fighter pilots who have LASIK get wavefront-guided, all-laser LASIK. NASA agrees, too—their astronauts undergo the same type of LASIK procedure.

Undergoing the LASIK Procedure

On the day of your LASIK procedure, it is natural to experience both excitement and nervousness. Understanding LASIK and trusting your surgeon are important to helping you feel confident, calm, and prepared on the day of your procedure. Each center does LASIK differently. In the paragraphs that follow, we describe how LASIK is done at our center.

Before the Procedure

You will need to arrange for someone to drive you to the surgery center and pick you up when you're ready to leave. You won't be able to drive immediately after the procedure because your vision will be blurry for a while. You should plan to spend about two hours at the center.

Wear comfortable clothing the day of your surgery. Do not wear makeup, skin moisturizer, perfume, or cologne because LASIK requires clean, sterile conditions. If you usually use makeup, use makeup remover to be sure all mascara and eyeliner are removed; you don't want these contaminants getting into your eye during surgery.

LASIK is performed while you are awake. You can't be put to sleep under anesthesia because we need you to look straight ahead during the laser treatment. To reduce your anxiety, we offer you an oral sedative, similar to Valium. You don't need to take it if you aren't nervous.

How the Procedure Is Performed

Before the surgery begins, your face is cleaned with a disinfectant, and a surgical cap is placed over your hair. You are given eyedrops to numb the eyes, which may sting for

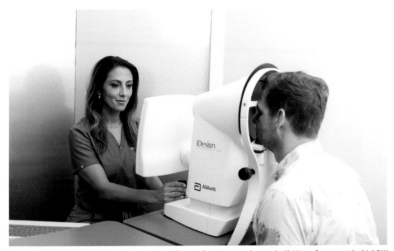

A wavefront analyzer measures hundreds of imperfections on the eyeball. Wavefront-guided LASIK produces sharper vision and a quicker recovery time.

a few seconds. No needles nor injections are used. Once in the laser suite, you are positioned comfortably, lying on your back in a reclining chair. The surgeon talks to you throughout the procedure so you know what is happening and what to expect next.

More anesthetic drops are placed in your eyes to ensure they are completely numb. If you are having all-laser LASIK (which is the case for almost all of our patients), the surgeon first places a gentle suction ring on the sclera to hold the eye motionless while the flap is made. You feel a mild pressure when this ring is placed on your eye. The laser flap maker is then lowered into contact with the suction ring, blocking your vision. You can't see for thirty seconds while the flap is made, which can be scary. This is normal. The suction ring is then removed and the flap is made on the other eye the same way. The surgeon then swings your reclining chair under the excimer laser. A small retainer, called an *eyelid speculum,* props open your eyelids to keep you from closing them during the procedure. The eyelid speculum does not hurt.

The surgeon gently lifts the hinged flap and proceeds to apply the laser to correct your vision. This usually takes twenty to ninety seconds per eye. You do not feel any pain as the laser sculpts the cornea by vaporizing small amounts of tissue. You

The LASIK Procedure

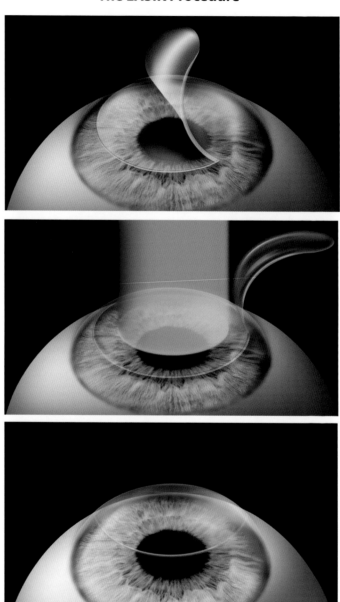

Figure 18. Top: A LASIK procedure begins with the surgeon using a laser to make a flap on the surface of the cornea, providing access to the cornea tissues underneath. *Middle:* Using an excimer laser, the surgeon reshapes the exposed cornea, correcting vision. *Bottom:* After the cornea is reshaped, the corneal flap is replaced; it stays in place without sutures.

hear a clicking or buzzing sound with each pulse of the laser while the surgeon is reshaping your cornea to correct your vision *(Figure 18)*.

While the sculpting is taking place, the surgeon will ask you to look at a small red light straight in front of you. You should focus on this light, but if you have trouble seeing it, don't worry. The laser has a tracking device that follows your eye during the laser treatment. The tracker provides an extra level of safety. If you move your eye during the treatment, the laser follows your eye, so the treatment is still applied in exactly the right location.

After the cornea is reshaped, the surgeon rinses the surface of the eye an then carefully replaces the corneal flap in its original position. The eye creates a natural vacuum that holds down the flap. The flap adheres like Velcro, so no sutures are necessary. The eyelid speculum is removed. You are now able to blink normally. The whole process takes five to six minutes per eye.

Your vision is hazy at first, but you immediately notice that it is improved compared to before LASIK. You can read a clock across the room. You sit with your eyes closed for about thirty minutes. Then your eyes are examined one more time to ensure that the corneal flap is properly positioned.

Immediately after surgery, your vision is somewhat blurred and hazy, similar to looking through dirty glasses. You may experience some burning or a gritty feeling in your eyes, which may last up to six hours. We give you a sedative to take when you get home. It is best to have your eyes closed for the first few hours after surgery, and sleep is the easiest way to accomplish this. After your nap, the discomfort is usually gone.

Upon awakening the next morning, you will typically experience a dramatic improvement in vision. Most people see well enough to drive to their next-day checkup.

Recovering from LASIK

For the first week or two after surgery, you will probably experience an intermittent feeling of grittiness in the eye. You are feeling the edge of the flap while it is healing. Lubricating eyedrops will help relieve this feeling. You may also notice that your eyes feel drier after LASIK, particularly when you

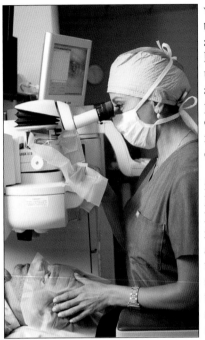

For LASIK surgery, you will be sedated but will remain awake. The procedure takes five to six minutes per eye.

wake up or toward the end of the day. Lubricating eyedrops, also called *artificial tears,* will help with this feeling, which usually resolves by six months after surgery. Although many patients initially notice halos or starburst around lights at night, these symptoms usually disappear within six months.

Most patients are genuinely surprised by how quickly their vision improves after LASIK. Although the corneal flap adheres quickly, your eyesight will fluctuate for a while until it finally reaches a point at which it becomes stable. The time it takes to establish visual stability after LASIK is usually one to three months.

Patients who have hyperopic LASIK (farsightedness treatment) may notice that at first their near vision is better than their distance vision. This is quite common, and the distance vision will continue to improve during the first month.

Until your vision stabilizes, you may feel more comfortable with a pair of eyeglasses to assist you with critical distance vision activities, such as driving at night. Patients over forty-five years of age will require a thin pair of glasses for reading, unless a monovision correction was done.

Postoperative Care

You will receive various eyedrops, including anti-inflammatory drops to promote healing and lubricating eyedrops. The surgeon's staff will instruct you in how to use them. Within hours of your surgery, constantly regenerating cells will already be growing over the edge of the corneal flap, helping to "glue" it down. This process takes a few hours. Avoid rubbing your eyes on the day of surgery. The corneal flap needs time to adhere evenly without being disturbed. Over the next several months, internal healing processes will totally seal the flap.

Keeping your follow-up appointments is important, even if your vision is perfect. Your doctor needs to monitor your healing to be sure it is normal.

Resuming Activities

Don't drive on the day of surgery. Resume driving only when your vision is clear enough that you are safe on the road. Most people easily see well enough to drive safely the morning after surgery, but some people require a few days before they feel comfortable enough to drive.

Avoid swimming, surfing, and hot tubs for one week to prevent contact with unwanted germs that could cause infection before the corneal flap has totally healed. Showers and baths are fine. Avoid dusty or smoky environments for three days after surgery.

It is fine to wear makeup, but avoid wearing mascara and eyeliner. Old mascara and eyeliner can accumulate germs, which you do not want to introduce into your eyes. If you wish to wear mascara or eyeliner during the first week after LASIK, use a new tube.

Results You Can Expect from LASIK

What are my chances of achieving 20/20 vision with LASIK? Can something bad happen to me during surgery? Every patient wants to know the answers to these questions.

Be aware that 20/20 vision or better is the likely outcome in everyone who has LASIK, but the exact chance of achieving 20/20 vision depends on your degree of correction. Although your doctor can't guarantee 20/20 eyesight after vision correction surgery, it is reasonable for you to ask your doctor to predict your chances for a successful outcome.

LASIK is a very safe procedure. *See* the Potential Complications section later in this chapter for any concerns you may have about the surgery.

What Is an Enhancement Procedure?

If you don't achieve 20/20 vision after LASIK, your doctor should recommend an *enhancement procedure* to you, if you wish. An enhancement procedure means doing a small amount of additional LASIK to improve your vision further. This is usually done three months after the original LASIK. Enhancement LASIK is even easier than the original LASIK procedure. Because you already have a flap, the doctor doesn't need to make a flap again. You return to the procedure room, where the doctor lifts the flap, applies a small amount of additional laser treatment, and replaces the flap. The recovery is usually faster than the initial LASIK treatment.

Generally speaking, if your vision is 20/20, we don't do enhancement procedures to try to get your vision to a super vision 20/15 level. However, there are exceptions. We like to say that the goal of surgery is to produce a smile. If you are 20/20 and not yet happy with your vision, if appropriate, we'll offer you an enhancement to correct your vision to 20/15.

The statistics we give below are typical results of the initial LASIK surgery, without considering enhancements. They are the results you can expect in the hands of an experienced surgeon—someone who has done at least 5,000 LASIK procedures. If enhancements were included, the results would look even better.

Tracking Statistics

Each surgeon achieves somewhat different results with the same laser and the same procedure. The best surgeons track their own results and adjust the laser to optimize each patient's outcome based on the surgeon's personal results. The reality is that most surgeons have not compiled personal statistics for one of three reasons: first, they haven't done enough procedures; second, they aren't willing to do the labor-intensive work of entering large numbers of cases into a database; or third, they don't have the statistical knowledge necessary to analyze their results. This is unfortunate because it reduces your chances of achieving 20/20 vision or better.

A surgeon who tracks his own results will give you a better chance of perfect vision and can also better educate you about what result you can expect, based on your degree of refractive error.

The percentage of people who achieve 20/40 vision is a key target that many surgeons use because 20/40 vision is good enough to drive legally without eyeglasses or contacts.

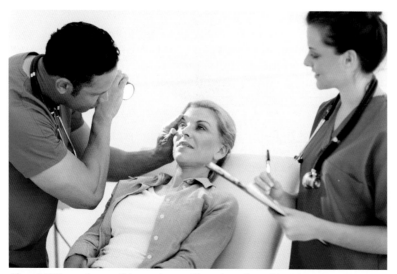

After a LASIK procedure, you'll be sent home with eyedrops that will both lubricate your eyes and prevent inflammation. Your surgeon will examine you the day after your LASIK procedure.

We don't believe that 20/40 vision is good enough, so we always strive for 20/20 vision or better.

Statistical Outcomes According to Your Refraction

Your chance of achieving 20/20 vision depends on how nearsighted or farsighted you are. To determine this, find your degree of myopia or hyperopia from a recent eyeglass or contact lens prescription, as discussed in chapter 1.

The statistics listed give you an indication of the results to expect from wavefront-guided laser treatment by an experienced surgeon. Keep in mind that the patients who did not achieve 20/20 vision without glasses are still seeing very well, almost always better than 20/40. They can do most things without eyeglasses or contacts, including driving a car. And if they wish to fine-tune their vision, an enhancement procedure can be done.

Mild Myopia

You have mild nearsightedness if the sphere part of your eyeglass prescription is between 0.00 and –3.00 diopters. A patient with mild myopia has a better than 97 percent chance of achieving 20/20 vision on the first procedure, and if enhancements are included, it rises to above 99 percent.

Moderate Myopia

You have moderate myopia if the sphere part of your eyeglass prescription is between –3.00 and –7.00 diopters. After the initial procedure, about 95 percent achieve 20/20 vision or better. Including enhancement surgery, 99 percent see 20/20 or better.

High Myopia

You have high myopia if the sphere part of your eyeglass prescription is between –7.00 and –10.00 diopters. Patients with high myopia have a 90 percent chance of seeing 20/20 or better. Including enhancement surgeries, they have a greater than 97 percent chance of seeing 20/20 or better.

Extreme Myopia

If the sphere part of your eyeglass prescription is more than –10.00, you have extreme myopia. Many patients with extreme myopia do well with LASIK, but we do not consider them optimal candidates. LASIK patients in this range are more likely to have enhancements and more likely to have problems with quality of vision, such as starburst, halos, or hazy vision. Patients in this group need to thoroughly discuss the risks and benefits of LASIK, as well as other options, with their doctor. Although enhancement rates are higher in this group of patients, because of other variables in the eye, there may be limitations on what can be done. These patients are often better candidates for the implantable contact lens, discussed in chapter 7.

Low and Moderate Hyperopia

If the sphere part of your eyeglass prescription is a positive number, you have farsightedness, or hyperopia. If the number is between +0.25 and +3.00, you have a low to moderate level of hyperopia. After your initial LASIK procedure, you have a 90 percent chance of achieving 20/20 vision.

Patients treated for hyperopia should be aware that their healing time will be slightly longer than for patients with myopia, and the chance that they will need an enhancement is somewhat higher. These numbers will vary according to the patient's original prescription, as well as the skill and experience level of the surgeon.

High Hyperopia

If the sphere part of your eyeglass prescription is more than +3.00, you have a high degree of hyperopia. For patients with high hyperopia, the results of LASIK are less predictable, and quality of vision may not be as good as for lower degrees of hyperopia. If you have hyperopia of more than +3.00 diopters, we generally do not recommend LASIK for you; you should instead consider refractive lens exchange, discussed in chapter 8.

Astigmatism

As explained earlier, astigmatism is the second number on your eyeglass prescription for each eye. Patients with mild astigmatism (less than 1.50 diopters) can expect outcomes and enhancement percentages nearly identical to those patients with myopia or hyperopia only. The presence of a greater degree of preoperative astigmatism will somewhat reduce your chance of achieving 20/20 vision after the initial procedure, making it more likely that you will have an enhancement. Also, astigmatism of more than 2.00 diopters somewhat increases your chance of getting starburst around lights at night. Astigmatism of 4.00 diopters or less can be corrected with LASIK.

Potential Complications with LASIK

Just as all surgical procedures carry risks, so does the LASIK procedure. However, when LASIK is performed by an experienced surgeon, the risk of complications is quite low. In fact, this surgery is among the safest procedures today when performed properly.

Many complications are preventable, either by proper preoperative evaluation or by expert surgical technique. An inexperienced surgeon may fail to detect a condition that would make you a poor candidate for LASIK, whereas an experienced surgeon may detect a contraindication and advise you not to have LASIK, or perhaps advise you to have a different procedure. There are many reasons to turn down a patient.

We've listed below both the rare and serious complications and the less rare and mild ones. Although this list is not exhaustive, it includes the possible complications that you need to know about in order to make an informed decision about proceeding with LASIK surgery.

Undercorrection

Undercorrection means that your refractive error wasn't fully corrected by LASIK. If you were nearsighted before surgery, it means you are still a little bit nearsighted afterward. A slight undercorrection will not seriously affect your vision and may even be desirable in nearsighted patients over forty to help with their reading vision. If the undercorrection is enough to cause significant blurring of vision, we recommend an enhancement procedure for you.

Overcorrection

Overcorrection means that your refractive error was corrected more than intended. If you were initially nearsighted, overcorrection means that you are farsighted after LASIK, making it hard to see clearly up close. If you were farsighted before LASIK, an overcorrection would make you nearsighted. In this case, your distance vision would be somewhat blurred and your near vision rather good.

An initial, temporary overcorrection is not uncommon, and usually rights itself in the first month as the eye heals. Patients can manage a temporary overcorrection by wearing glasses until the problem resolves. As with undercorrection, a significant overcorrection can be treated with an enhancement procedure, after your vision has stabilized.

Dry Eye

LASIK makes the eyes somewhat drier than before surgery, usually for the first few months. For most patients this is not a problem because the eyes have more moisture than needed, so a little dryness is not bothersome. However, in rare cases patients develop more significant dryness after LASIK. These patients experience dryness throughout the day. You are more at risk for this condition if you have dry eyes before LASIK while wearing glasses. (Many people have dry eyes while wearing contact lenses, but these people are usually excellent candidates for LASIK because the eyes can be much more comfortable after LASIK than with contacts.) An important part of the comprehensive examination is an evaluation of your tears to ensure that your chance of experiencing post-LASIK dryness is minimal.

If you develop significant dryness, a variety of treatments are now available. These include taking dietary supplements, using lubricating eyedrops, using prescription eyedrops that improve tear production, and blocking your tear drainage canals with tiny plugs to retain more tears in your eyes.

Corneal Abrasion

The eye is covered by a thin layer of skin, called the epithelium. This skin is just like the skin on your hand except that it is clear so you can see through it. Occasionally, the minor trauma of surgery causes part of the epithelium to slough off. This is called a *corneal abrasion* or *corneal epithelial defect*, and occurs in about 2 percent of LASIK patients. This doesn't harm your eye and doesn't interfere with the laser treatment. Your eye will feel scratchy for a few days while the epithelium heals. Abrasions always heal, usually in one to three days.

Nighttime Starburst and Halos

All people, whether or not they have had LASIK, experience some starburst or halos at night. These night-vision disturbances occur when you are in a dark environment and look at a small bright light, such as a headlight or a streetlight. *Halo* is the glow that surrounds the light source, and starburst is little spiky rays of light that emanate from the light source. Starbursts and halos occur because the pupil dilates in low-light conditions. The dilated pupil allows more peripheral light rays (rays coming in from the sides) to enter the eye. These rays are more likely to scatter, instead of coming to a precise focus. You perceive the scattered light as starburst or halos. Look carefully at a headlight or streetlight tonight so you understand what we're talking about. Incidentally, this scattering of light is why everyone notices that their night vision is not as good as their daytime vision.

Some patients experience an increase in starburst and halo after LASIK. These symptoms can be bothersome in dim light conditions, such as driving at night. Starburst and halo improve gradually, and the overwhelming majority of significant starburst problems disappear on their own by six months. However, if you still have significant starburst or halos at six months, they tend to persist.

No one can predict whether you will get more starburst or halos after surgery, but we can tell you your odds. If you have high myopia or high astigmatism, you have more chance of noticing significant night-vision disturbances. In one FDA study that our center performed, about 10 percent of highly nearsighted people noticed halos all the time at night. This is a primary reason why we prefer the implantable contact lens for high levels of myopia. If you have a low or moderate correction, then significant night-vision disturbances are rare. Many eye doctors used to believe that patients with larger pupils had a greater chance of developing starburst or halos at night, but a number of major studies have now shown that this is not true.

If you develop significant starburst or halos after LASIK, there are treatment options. A light prescription for night driving can help, as can the use at dusk of eyedrops that reduce the size of your pupils. The newer wavefront-guided laser treatment has been shown to significantly reduce night-vision disturbances compared with conventional laser treatment, which is another reason we use wavefront-guided treatment in all eligible patients.

Problems with Quality of Vision

Rarely, patients after LASIK experience a slight decrease in quality of vision. Vision can seem slightly dirty or hazy, like wearing glasses or contacts that aren't clean. Vision tends to improve over time. This complication is very rare except in those with very high levels of nearsightedness or astigmatism. This is another reason we prefer the implantable contacts lens for extreme myopia.

Corneal Flap Complications

The older microkeratome blade can occasionally cut the flap incorrectly. The flap can be left too small, too thin, detached, or have a hole in the middle. If this happens the surgeon will abort the operation and replace the flap. This complication is extremely rare with all-laser LASIK, which is another reason we only offer all-laser LASIK over the microkeratome blade.

Striae

Rarely, the corneal flap may shift slightly in the first twelve hours after LASIK surgery. If the flap shifts slightly, wrinkles form, just as wrinkles form in a carpet if you step on it and it isn't properly nailed down. The medical term for these wrinkles is *striae*. If striae are present in the center of the cornea, they may blur your vision. You will be asked to keep your eyes closed and not to rub your eyes for the first few hours after surgery, which helps prevent the flap from shifting.

Fortunately, striae are easy to fix with a short procedure. The flap is lifted and laid back down smoothly. The surgeon places a special, clear contact lens, called a bandage contact lens, over your eye to hold the flap securely in place overnight.

Epithelial Ingrowth

The cornea is covered by a thin, clear skin, called epithelium. This clear skin is made of epithelial cells. When the LASIK flap is lifted and replaced, these cells normally grow back over the top of the flap. Rarely, the cells grow under the flap instead. This condition is called *epithelial ingrowth*. These cells can cause blurred vision or irritation. Epithelial ingrowth is easy to treat if detected early by gently lifting the flap and clearing away the trapped epithelial cells. Detecting epithelial ingrowth is one of the reasons why it is important that you return for your scheduled follow-up visits.

Corneal Ectasia

We have already noted that keratoconus makes you a poor candidate for LASIK. *Corneal ectasia* is what we call keratoconus that develops after LASIK. It is very rare. Some patients develop ectasia because the surgeon was too aggressive in removing tissue during the procedure. Some patients with ectasia after LASIK have keratoconus that should have been detected preoperatively but wasn't. This is one of the reasons a careful preoperative exam is so important.

Rarely, some people develop ectasia after a LASIK procedure that was done properly where was no evidence of keratoconus in the preoperative exam. It appears that these rare individuals had subclinical keratoconus before surgery. *Subclinical* means it was present but not detectable. In some of these individuals, the LASIK flap seems to accelerate the underlying disease. In others, it appears they would have developed keratoconus even without LASIK surgery because of their genetic predisposition.

Corneal ectasia is rare in anyone, but less rare in young people with high corrections and thin corneas. In those patients at risk of ectasia, we may recommend PRK or the implantable contact lens instead.

Ectasia and keratoconus can now be arrested with a procedure called *corneal crosslinking*. In corneal crosslinking, the cornea is saturated with riboflavin, a vitamin, which is then exposed to ultraviolet (UV) light. The combination of the UV light and the riboflavin cause the fibers in the cornea to bond together; this action strengthens the cornea and stops the progression of the disease.

Infection and Other Potential Serious Complications

Infection is extremely rare after LASIK, occurring in about 1 in 10,000 surgeries done by an experienced surgeon. It is a feared complication because an infection can cause a scar in the cornea, leading to blurred vision. The good news is that infection is much more rare with LASIK than with contact lenses, so from the point of view of this serious complication, LASIK is safer than contact lenses.

As with any surgery, proper technique is the best way to avoid infection. If your eye does become infected, this will likely occur during the first forty-eight to seventy-two hours after LASIK. This is why it is so important for the first week to avoid any contact with substances that carry bacteria, such as old eye makeup, hot tubs, and swimming pools. It is also essential to go to all of your follow-up visits, even if everything seems fine. You may be prescribed antibiotic eyedrops after surgery to prevent infection.

Any surgery can result in loss of vision. Fortunately, this is extremely rare with LASIK. We have personally never had a patient lose their vision from LASIK. An important publication from the Oregon Health and Science University compared the risk of loss of vision from LASIK to the risk of loss of vision from contact lenses, and found that LASIK was the safer option. Nevertheless, you shouldn't be complacent. It is important to follow all the surgeon's instructions, both pre- and postoperatively, to make the LASIK procedure as safe as possible.

Frequently Asked Questions about LASIK

LASIK surgeons are accustomed to having patients ask many questions. An important part of our role is to educate you. Here are some of the questions we're asked most often.

Is LASIK painful?

No. Before the procedure begins, your eye is numbed with eyedrops. You may feel a mild sensation of pressure as the corneal flap is being made, but the procedure will not hurt at all. After the surgery, the minor discomfort you may experience will typically last only a few hours. Sleep and lubricating eyedrops, as well as acetaminophen or ibuprofen, are usually enough to take care of any discomfort. At our center, we also offer you a sleeping pill to allow you to sleep through any discomfort.

How long does the LASIK procedure take?

Most patients are pleasantly surprised at how quickly LASIK is performed. Expect an experienced surgeon to complete the procedure in five to six minutes per eye.

How long will it take for my eyes to heal?

The healing process is remarkably fast, with few associated side effects. Postoperative discomfort is quite minor. You may notice a burning or gritty sensation and watery eyes for up to six hours after surgery. Your eyes may feel irritated on and off for a week or two. Lubricating eyedrops alleviate this irritation. In terms of vision, more than 90 percent of our patients see 20/20 or better the day after surgery.

What happens if my vision isn't clear enough after LASIK?

Even in the hands of a skilled surgeon, each person's eyes respond differently to the excimer laser, both during the surgery and while healing. Not everyone gets perfect vision. About 5 percent of LASIK patients find their vision isn't as clear as they hoped. In this situation we will usually recommend an enhancement procedure. For an enhancement procedure, the surgeon gently lifts the preexisting flap and performs a small additional laser treatment. Recovery time is similar to that of the original procedure. If you do need an enhancement procedure, you must wait for your eye to stabilize. We typically do enhancements three months after the original procedure.

An enhancement procedure can also be done years later if your eyesight changes over time.

How long will the correction last?

Once your eyes have stabilized, usually in three months or less, your vision correction is permanent. Unless you had a monovision correction, you will eventually need eyeglasses for reading as you age, just like everyone else with good vision.

Although LASIK doesn't wear off, your vision can change during your lifetime. LASIK doesn't prevent your eyes from changing if they would have changed anyway. If your vision does change when you are older, an enhancement procedure can usually be done to restore excellent vision without glasses.

Will I be able to drive immediately after LASIK?

You can't drive the day of surgery because you will have blurry vision and may have taken a sedative. By the next morning, however, almost everyone can drive safely. You should use your own good judgment before you start driving again.

When can I go back to work?

Most people return to work the day after LASIK. We've even had patients work a night shift after their afternoon LASIK procedure. If you work in a very dusty environment, such as a construction site, wait a couple of days before going back to work.

Although most patients can function normally at work the day after surgery, your vision may still be somewhat blurry and your eyes may be occasionally irritated, so we recommend that you not schedule any critical appointments or meetings for that day.

If I have dry eyes, will it affect my LASIK surgery?

That depends. Many people have LASIK because they have mild dry eyes and cannot wear contact lenses comfortably. These patients are delighted to have good vision without the irritation of contacts. On the other hand, if you have moderate or severe dry eyes, LASIK may not be a good idea. Part of your comprehensive preoperative exam will be to evaluate your eyes for dryness and alert you if there are any abnormalities found. Sometimes dry eyes can be treated preoperatively and you can still have successful LASIK.

LASIK

If I've had previous eye surgery, am I still a candidate for LASIK?

Often, people who have had previous eye surgery are candidates for LASIK. However, these can be more difficult surgeries and have less predictable results. For example, LASIK has been used following an older form of refractive surgery, radial keratotomy (RK). With RK, the cornea is flattened by making small, spokelike incisions around its periphery to correct myopia and astigmatism. LASIK following RK can succeed so long as the patient's vision is relatively stable and there is not significant corneal scarring in the incisions.

If I have thin corneas, am I still a candidate for LASIK?

Often, yes, depending on your degree of correction. If your cornea is thin, removing the amount of tissue necessary to treat a high degree of myopia may weaken your cornea. The surgeon will calculate the amount of tissue to be removed. If too much tissue will need to be removed, to ensure your cornea is not weakened the surgeon should recommend PRK or an implantable contact lens instead.

Can I wear contact lenses after surgery, if needed?

After surgery, if you still need correction in one or both eyes, you may elect to wear contact lenses. If you tolerated the contacts before LASIK, it is likely you will tolerate them afterward. In practice, though, rather than returning you to contact lens wear, your surgeon should recommend an enhancement to sharpen your vision.

Could the LASIK procedure cause problems years from now?

Unknown complications years down the road are very unlikely. LASIK is a form of lamellar refractive surgery, a type of surgery that has been performed since 1949. People who have undergone earlier types of lamellar refractive surgery—much less accurate and more invasive than LASIK—have not developed unexpected problems during the past fifty years.

Will having LASIK prevent eye diseases?

No. LASIK does not prevent cataracts, glaucoma, retinal detachment, macular degeneration, or any other eye disease. That is why it is important to still have regular eye checkups after LASIK, even if your vision is perfect. If you are diagnosed with a disease in the future, LASIK will not affect its treatment.

Should I have surgery on both eyes at the same time?

Some patients choose to have one eye treated at a time because they worry, "What if something goes wrong?" These patients can have the other eye done as soon as the next day. Most patients do both eyes on the same day. We are extremely confident about the safety of LASIK. No one in our practice has lost vision in either one or both eyes from the procedure. Having both eyes done together avoids making two trips to the surgery center and speeds the recovery. Correcting the eyes on separate days leaves you with an interim period of imbalanced vision during which only one eye is corrected. In the end, the choice is yours, and you should feel no pressure to do it one way or the other.

Should I wait for the next generation of LASIK treatment?

LASIK is a fairly stable technology now, with advances happening incrementally. In general, we are all aging faster than LASIK is getting better. With the all-laser wavefront-guided technology now available, waiting longer doesn't make much sense.

6

PRK

The procedure that originally made wide use of the excimer laser was photorefractive keratectomy, abbreviated *PRK,* first performed in 1987. Like LASIK, PRK is a refractive surgical procedure that uses an excimer laser to reshape the cornea. However, rather than creating a flap, as in LASIK, and then reshaping the deeper corneal layers, PRK uses the excimer laser to sculpt directly on the surface of the cornea. In PRK, the epithelium (the clear skin covering the surface of the cornea) is removed. This exposes the stroma. The laser then sculpts away the stromal tissue to correct your vision *(Figure 19).* The epithelium grows back to cover the cornea again over the next three to four days.

You can think of PRK as LASIK without the flap. The message of this chapter is that PRK and LASIK are very similar. Rather than duplicate much of the material in the LASIK chapter, we refer back to that chapter frequently in this chapter on PRK. If you skipped the chapter on LASIK and came directly here, we recommend you go back and read the LASIK chapter first.

Yet there are differences between PRK and LASIK, the main one being that PRK has a slower recovery than LASIK. Your eye will often be sore for three or four days after surgery while it heals. We give our PRK patients numbing eyedrops to take home to use if their eye hurts. Your vision will be fairly blurry for about a week while the epithelium heals, and perfect vision often takes a month or longer to achieve. In the long run, though, the results of PRK and LASIK are the same because they are very similar procedures performed with the same laser. In general, our patients prefer LASIK for the faster

The PRK Procedure

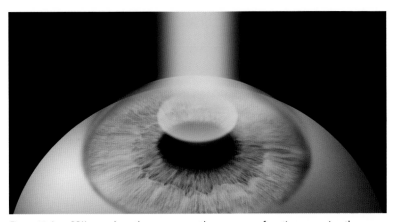

Figure 19. In a PRK procedure, the surgeon gently removes surface tissue covering the cornea rather than making a flap. Then, the excimer laser sculpts the cornea, to correct nearsightedness, farsightedness, or astigmatism.

recovery. We reserve PRK for those people who aren't optimal candidates for LASIK.

PRK is referred to by a number of different names. If you search the Internet, you'll find it called *flapless LASIK, epi-LASIK, surface ablation,* or *LASEK.* We prefer PRK, and will use that term in this book.

How PRK Corrects Your Vision

During the PRK procedure, the outermost layer of the cornea, the epithelium, is removed, exposing the stromal tissue beneath. The exposed stromal tissue is then precisely sculpted by a laser into a new shape to correct your vision. Doing PRK on your eyes is analogous to sculpting a contact lens onto the surface of your eye: you see clearly, but without the hassle of removing, cleaning, or changing a contact lens anymore.

PRK and Myopic Correction

As explained in chapter 1, patients who are nearsighted have corneas with too much curvature in proportion to the length of their eyes. The excimer laser reshapes the underlying stroma by removing more tissue from the center of the cornea than from the periphery. The result is a flatter cornea with less focusing power. The surgeon's precise measurements are programmed into the computer to guide the excimer laser. The result is that light rays coming through the cornea now come to a point of focus on the retina rather than in front of it.

PRK and Hyperopic Correction

Farsighted patients have corneas that are not curved enough for the length of their eyes. The excimer laser is programmed to remove tissue predominantly from the periphery of the cornea, leaving the center of the cornea untouched; this creates more of a domed shape. The increased curvature of the cornea allows light rays to focus on the retina rather than behind it.

PRK and Astigmatism

To treat astigmatism, the excimer laser removes tissue in an oval shape, correcting the shape of the cornea in one direction more than the other. The goal is to eliminate the oval shape of the corneal surface so that light rays passing through the cornea meet at a single point of focus on the retina. Astigmatism can be corrected with the laser in combination with nearsightedness or farsightedness.

Are You a Candidate for PRK?

With few exceptions, if you are a good candidate for LASIK, you are a good candidate for PRK. Conversely, if you are a poor candidate for LASIK because of thin corneas or keratoconus, you may still be a good candidate for PRK. This section will cover who is and who isn't a good candidate for PRK.

The following conditions can affect whether or not you are a candidate for PRK.

Thin Cornea

The major benefit of PRK is that it can be performed on patients with thin corneas. LASIK involves lifting a flap and then beginning the laser treatment in the middle layers of the cornea. In PRK, the laser treatment starts on the surface of the cornea, just below the epithelium, so PRK doesn't penetrate as deeply into the cornea. That is a better option if your cornea is thin.

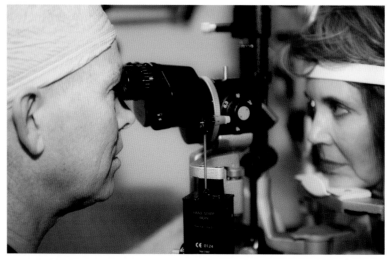

Your ophthalmologist will monitor your progress for several months after a PRK procedure. It typically takes two to three months for your vision to fully stabilize, but most patients see a major improvement the day after the procedure.

Degree of Refractive Error

The best candidates for PRK have an eyeglass prescription that isn't extreme. This means, if you are nearsighted, you may have myopia of up to −8.00 diopters. If you are farsighted, your hyperopia may be up to +3.00 diopters. Your level of astigmatism may be as high as +4.00 diopters. Patients outside of these ranges can still have PRK, but they require a large degree of corneal reshaping and expectations for crisp, clear vision are lower. Above −8.00 diopters of myopia, we usually recommend the implantable contact lens. Above +3.00 diopters of hyperopia, we prefer refractive lens exchange. Both of these options are covered in detail in later chapters.

Keratoconus

As described in chapter 6, keratoconus is an uncommon, hereditary condition that weakens the cornea. Keratoconus progresses gradually in younger people and then stabilizes around the age of forty. We don't do LASIK on patients with keratoconus because the flap can accelerate the weakening of the cornea. Because PRK doesn't penetrate as deeply into the cornea as LASIK and doesn't require a flap, PRK is a better procedure for people with this condition. That isn't to say that people with keratoconus are often good candidates for PRK, however. That depends on a variety of factors that your doctor will need to address at your comprehensive preoperative examination.

Cataract

Just as with LASIK, if you have a cataract, you are not a good candidate for PRK. You are probably a good candidate for refractive lens exchange (covered in detail in chapter 8) because refractive lens exchange corrects both the vision and the cataract.

Basement Membrane Dystrophy

Basement membrane dystrophy is a hereditary condition that causes the epithelium, the clear skin that covers the cornea, to slough off spontaneously, resulting in a corneal abrasion. It is a relative contraindication for LASIK. Sometimes, PRK is a reasonable approach in patients with this condition because removing the epithelium is actually a treatment for basement membrane dystrophy. Your eye surgeon will advise you if PRK is a good option for you.

Prior Episodes of Herpes Infection of the Cornea

Prior episodes of herpes infection of cornea are a contraindication for PRK because the removal of the epithelium can stimulate a reactivation of the virus.

Significant Dry Eye

PRK makes the eyes drier to the same degree as LASIK does, so patients who start with significantly dry eyes can be uncomfortable after PRK. (PRK and dry eye is discussed in more detail later in this chapter.) On the other hand, mild dry eye can make contact lens wear very uncomfortable. Such people often do much better with PRK than with contact lenses. The surgeon will evaluate your tear production and advise you if PRK is a good alternative for you.

Although the conditions listed are generally contraindications to PRK, many are not absolute contraindications. If you have one of these conditions, consultation with an experienced PRK surgeon will help you determine whether PRK is still a possibility for you.

Seeing Better than 20/20 with PRK

We have already discussed in chapter 5 how you can achieve better than 20/20 vision with wavefront-guided LASIK. We use the same wavefront-guided method for PRK. We use a wavefront analyzer to measure the imperfections of your vision objectively at 1,200 different points in your eye. This information is fed into the laser, which then customizes a slightly different correction at each point of your eye to eliminate the imperfections. The result for many people is better than 20/20 vision with PRK.

Undergoing the PRK Procedure

On the day of your PRK procedure, it is natural to experience both excitement and nervousness. Understanding PRK and trusting your surgeon are important to helping you feel confident, calm, and prepared on the day of your procedure. Each vision correction center does PRK differently. In the paragraphs that follow, we describe how PRK is done at our center.

Before the Procedure

You will need to arrange for someone to drive you to the surgery center and pick you up when you're ready to leave. You won't be able to drive immediately after the procedure because your vision will be blurry. You should plan to spend about two hours at the center.

Wear comfortable clothing the day of your surgery. Do not wear makeup, skin moisturizer, perfume, or cologne because PRK requires clean, sterile conditions. If you usually use makeup, use makeup remover to be sure all mascara and eyeliner are removed; you don't want these contaminants getting into your eye during surgery.

PRK is performed while you are awake. You can't be put to sleep under anesthesia because we need you to look straight ahead during the laser treatment. To reduce your anxiety, you will be offered an oral sedative, like Valium. You don't need to take it if you aren't nervous.

How the Procedure Is Performed

Before the surgery begins, your face is cleaned with a disinfectant, and a surgical cap is placed over your hair. You are given eyedrops to numb the eyes. Once in the surgical suite, you are positioned comfortably, lying on your back in a reclining chair. The surgeon talks to you throughout the procedure so you know what to expect next.

More anesthetic eyedrops are placed in your eye to be sure your eye is completely numb. No injections or needles are used. A small retainer, called an eyelid speculum, props open your eyelids to keep you from closing them during the procedure. The eyelid speculum does not hurt.

The surgeon gently removes the epithelium, which is the layer of clear skin that covers the cornea. The epithelium must be removed because it blocks the laser from reshaping the stroma. This step differs from the initial step of LASIK surgery, during which the flap is pulled back from the surface to expose the deeper layers of the cornea.

Next, the surgeon will use the laser to sculpt your cornea, enabling light to focus properly on the retina. PRK, like LASIK, is performed with an excimer laser, which reshapes the cornea with its cool, pulsing beam of ultraviolet light. This part of the procedure takes twenty to ninety seconds. As the laser removes tissue and reshapes the cornea, you will hear a tapping noise, which is caused by the laser energy.

While the sculpting is taking place, the surgeon will ask you to look at a small red light straight in front of you. You should focus on this light, but if you have trouble seeing it, don't worry. The laser has a tracking device that follows your eye during the laser treatment. The tracker provides an extra level of safety. If you move your eye during the treatment, the laser follows your eye, so the treatment is still applied in exactly the right location.

Once the procedure is complete, a special, clear contact lens, called a bandage contact lens, is placed over your eye to help keep you more comfortable while the corneal epithelium grows back, usually in three to four days. A typical PRK procedure takes about five minutes per eye.

After the procedure, your vision is hazy, but you immediately notice that it is improved compared to before PRK. You can read a clock across the room. You sit with your eyes closed for about twenty minutes. Your eyes are examined one more time to ensure that the bandage contact lenses are properly positioned, and you are on your way home.

Recovering from PRK

Healing after PRK happens in two phases. The first phase is the healing of the epithelium over the area of laser treatment, which takes three or four days. During this phase the eyes can be uncomfortable and the vision is blurry. The second phase begins when the epithelium heals. During this phase the eye is comfortable but the vision is still blurry.

Managing Discomfort

During PRK the epithelium was removed from the center of your cornea. The epithelium is a clear skin, and its absence is uncomfortable, just as the absence of skin from your fingertip is uncomfortable. While the epithelium is healing, you may have mild to moderate discomfort in your eyes. Typically, patients say that it feels as if they've scratched their eye or have a grain of sand in their eye. During this time, our efforts are directed at making sure you are comfortable. The bandage contact lens is very helpful in improving comfort because it acts like a bandage on the eye. One of the eyedrops you will take is a nonsteroidal anti-inflammatory agent, similar to ibuprofen. This is a good pain reliever. We also prescribe an oral pain reliever, such as Vicodin, though most people find they don't need it.

Finally, at least at our center, you will be given numbing eyedrops so you can numb your eyes at home if they start to hurt. These methods will keep your eyes comfortable after the PRK while the epithelium is healing.

After four days, the eyes are usually comfortable again, though the vision is still quite blurry. At this point the epithelium has completely healed over the area of the laser treatment. The bandage contact lens is then removed.

Achieving Good Vision

The second phase of recovery from PRK begins when the epithelium has healed. During this phase the eyes are comfortable but the vision is initially blurry. As this phase of recovery progresses, the vision gradually clears up.

During the first month after surgery, you will notice a gradual improvement in your vision. It is common to experience fluctuations in your vision during the first two to three weeks, especially for those with higher corrections. Your eyesight will continue to improve until it becomes stable. The time it takes

PRK

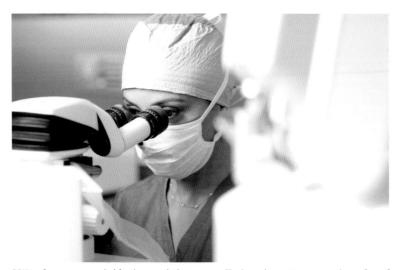

PRK is often recommended for those with thin corneas. The laser does not penetrate the surface of the eye as deeply as the laser used for LASIK.

to reach visual stability after PRK varies for each patient. For some, stability can be achieved in a few weeks. For others, stable vision may take three to six months.

Until your vision stabilizes, you may feel more comfortable with a thin pair of eyeglasses to assist you with critical distance vision activities, such as driving at night. Patients over forty-five years of age will require a thin pair of glasses for reading, unless a monovision correction was done.

At your consultation, you will have decided whether to have surgery on both eyes the same day or to have each eye treated on different days. With LASIK, we routinely do both eyes on the same day. With PRK, the return of clear vision is slower. If we do both eyes together, you will have blurry vision for a while in both eyes. If we do one eye at a time, you can rely on the vision in the unoperated-on eye while the blurry vision in the operated eye recovers. The major drawback to operating on one eye at a time is the inconvenience of going through the procedure and the recovery twice. Our experience is that most patients choose to do both eyes at the same time.

Postoperative Care

You will come into the office the day after your procedure for a checkup. You will return about five days later, once your corneal epithelium has healed, to have the bandage contact lens removed. Then you will typically be seen one and six months after surgery to ensure that healing is occurring properly. Six months after surgery your vision is usually completely stable.

You will use several different eyedrops. These include an antibiotic drop to prevent infection and a steroid drop to promote healing. As mentioned previously, you will also use a nonsteroidal anti-inflammatory eyedrop and the numbing drops as needed. The surgeon's staff will instruct you in how to use these drops.

It is fine to wear makeup, but avoid wearing old mascara and eyeliner for the first week after surgery. Old mascara and eyeliner can accumulate germs, which you do not want to introduce into your eyes. If you wish to wear mascara or eyeliner during the first week after surgery, open a fresh tube. For the same reason, avoid dusty environments until the contact lens bandage is removed. While the bandage contact lens is in your eyes, avoid rubbing your eyes; doing so could dislodge the lens.

Resuming Activities

Don't drive on the day of surgery. Resume driving only when your vision is clear enough that you are safe on the road. It may be a few days before you feel comfortable enough to drive, and even longer before you feel comfortable driving at night. Also, stay away from swimming pools, Jacuzzis, and hot tubs for at least a week after surgery. Bacteria in the water could cause an infection. It is fine to shower or bathe, though, because tap water has very few bacteria.

Otherwise, there are very few restrictions on your activities after your surgery. Reading, computer work, watching television, and flying are all fine to do immediately. You can restart your regular exercise regimen the morning after surgery.

Results You Can Expect from PRK

What are my chances of achieving 20/20 vision with PRK? Can something bad happen to me during surgery? These are the questions that every patient wants to ask.

Be aware that, although most PRK patients are already doing quite well at their one-month examination, it may take several months before we know if you achieved perfect vision. Often, patients who are severely nearsighted or farsighted must wait the longest for full results. The eye needs to heal fully before the doctor can actually determine the final result.

PRK Statistics

PRK is done using the same lasers and the same measurements as LASIK. The only difference between the PRK and LASIK procedures is the absence of the flap in PRK. Not surprisingly, the results of PRK and LASIK are the same, although getting to the final result takes longer with PRK. The great majority of people who have PRK achieve 20/20 vision or better. Your exact chance of achieving 20/20 vision depends on your degree of correction. Refer to the chapter on LASIK to determine your chance of getting 20/20 vision. The numbers there apply to PRK as well.

What Is an Enhancement Procedure?

If you don't achieve 20/20 vision after PRK, your doctor may recommend an enhancement procedure to you, if you wish. An enhancement procedure means doing a small amount of additional PRK to improve your vision further. During a PRK enhancement, the surface skin (the epithelium) is removed again, and you will experience another three to four days of mild to moderate discomfort. You will be prescribed medication to ease any discomfort. A minimum wait of six months after the original PRK is required for the eyes to become sufficiently stable for PRK enhancement.

Generally speaking, if your vision is 20/20, we don't do enhancement procedures to try to get your vision to a super vision 20/15 level. However, there are exceptions. We like to say that the goal of surgery is to produce a smile. If you are 20/20 and not yet happy with your vision, if appropriate, we'll offer you an enhancement to correct your vision to 20/15.

Potential Complications with PRK

In general, the complications of PRK and LASIK are very similar. Just as all surgical procedures carry risks, so does the PRK procedure. However, when PRK is performed by an experienced surgeon, the risk of complications is quite low. In fact, this surgery is among the safest procedures today when performed properly.

One advantage of PRK over LASIK is that there is no risk of flap complications because no corneal flap is created. Striae and epithelial ingrowth don't occur with PRK.

We've listed both the rare and serious complications and the less rare and mild ones. Although this list is not exhaustive, it includes the possible complications that you need to know about in order to be comfortable proceeding with PRK surgery.

Corneal Haze

Corneal haze is clouding of the cornea during the healing process. This clouding may cause blurry or hazy vision. As a general rule, the worse your eyesight was going into the procedure, the more you are at risk for developing corneal haze. Significant corneal haze following PRK is extremely rare with today's equipment and medications. Haze eventually disappears by itself, but this can take months or years. If it develops, corneal haze is usually re-treated with the laser to physically remove it, although this is necessary in fewer than 1 percent of patients.

Recurrent Erosions

During the PRK procedure, the epithelium is removed and then heals. Rarely after PRK, a small area of epithelium can slip off on its own. This usually happens at night during sleep or on awakening in the morning. When this happens, the eye hurts and waters for a few minutes to several hours. These small epithelial slips are called *recurrent erosions* and can recur over several weeks or months. Recurrent erosions can be treated with medicines or with a laser treatment.

Undercorrection

Undercorrection means that your refractive error wasn't fully corrected by PRK. If you were nearsighted before surgery, it means you are still a little bit nearsighted afterward. A slight undercorrection will not seriously affect your vision and may even be desirable in nearsighted patients over forty to help with their reading vision. If the undercorrection is enough to cause significant blurring of vision, we will recommend an enhancement procedure for you, generally after six months have passed.

Overcorrection

Overcorrection means that your refractive error was corrected more than intended. If you were initially nearsighted, overcorrection means that you are farsighted after PRK, making it hard to see clearly up close. If you were farsighted before PRK, an overcorrection would make you nearsighted. In this case, your distance vision would be somewhat blurred and your near vision rather good.

An initial, temporary overcorrection is not uncommon and usually rights itself in the first month as the eye heals. Patients can manage a temporary overcorrection by wearing glasses until the problem resolves. As with undercorrections, a significant overcorrection can be treated with an enhancement procedure. An enhancement for overcorrection is usually performed six months after the initial treatment, once your vision has stabilized.

Problems with Quality of Vision

Rarely, patients after PRK experience a slight decrease in quality of vision. Vision can seem slightly dirty or hazy, like wearing glasses or contacts that aren't clean. Vision tends to improve over time. This complication is very rare except in those with very high levels of nearsightedness or astigmatism. This is another reason we prefer implantable contacts lenses for extreme myopia.

Dry Eye

Just as with LASIK, PRK makes the eyes somewhat drier than before surgery, usually for the first few months. Some doctors think that PRK causes less dryness after LASIK so they recommend PRK to patients with dry eyes. That is not our experience. Our colleagues and we studied this question a decade ago and found no difference in postoperative dryness between PRK and LASIK. Other studies have similarly found no difference. We avoid both PRK and LASIK in patients with significant dryness preoperatively. The treatment of dryness after PRK is the same as with LASIK; refer to the LASIK chapter for a discussion of this.

Corneal Ectasia

Keratoconus is a hereditary weakness in the cornea that causes the cornea to bulge outward, causing blurred vision. When keratoconus develops after PRK or LASIK, we call it corneal ectasia. Corneal ectasia is rare in any case, but is less common after PRK. It may be that the LASIK flap slightly weakens a cornea already predisposed to bulging outward. PRK is the preferred procedure with someone in whom we are concerned about the possibility of ectasia after surgery.

Other Potential Complications

Starburst and halos at night can occur after PRK, just as they can after LASIK. Similarly, serious complications like infection can occur after PRK also, although very rarely. Refer to the section on these potential complications in the LASIK chapter.

Comparing PRK with LASIK

PRK and LASIK are performed with the same type of laser, and both procedures use the laser to reshape the eye in the same way. The difference between PRK and LASIK is that LASIK uses a flap and PRK doesn't.

Range of Correction

PRK and LASIK cover the same range of correction—low to moderate farsightedness and low to high nearsightedness, with or without astigmatism.

Depth of Penetration

Because no corneal flap is created, the depth of penetration of PRK into the cornea is less than with LASIK. PRK alters only the surface of the cornea. LASIK, on the other hand, penetrates into deeper layers of the cornea.

Recovery of Vision

The recovery from PRK is slower than with LASIK. After LASIK, your vision is usually 20/20 or close to it by the next morning. A week after PRK, average vision has improved to 20/40, and often takes a month or more to reach 20/20. If you have PRK completed in both eyes at the same time, you may need to take some additional time off work to let your vision sharpen up.

Discomfort

Because your eyes are numbed during surgery, you will feel no pain during either LASIK or PRK. Mild to moderate discomfort is typical with PRK during the first three or four days after surgery. The discomfort is caused by the absence of the epithelium and resolves as the new epithelium grows over the area of laser treatment. In LASIK, the epithelium is not removed, so postoperative discomfort usually lasts only about two to four hours.

Vision Outcome

The final visual results achieved by LASIK and PRK are the same, although it takes longer for the eye to heal completely with PRK. You achieve your final vision in PRK in one to six months, whereas with LASIK this typically occurs in one week to one month.

Frequently Asked Questions about PRK

PRK surgeons are accustomed to having patients ask many questions. An important part of our role as surgeons is to educate you. Here are some of the questions we are asked most often.

Is the PRK procedure painful?

No. The procedure is painless because the eye is completely numbed with anesthetic eyedrops. These drops are very effective, so no injections or IVs are needed. After the surgery, discomfort occurs on and off for three or four days. Surgeons typically prescribe an oral pain reliever for you. At our center, we also give you numbing eyedrops to take home to ensure that you are comfortable.

How long does the PRK procedure take?

Most patients are pleasantly surprised at how quickly PRK is performed. Expect an experienced surgeon to complete the procedure in five or six minutes per eye.

How long will it take for my eyes to heal?

The healing process for PRK takes longer than for LASIK because the epithelium is removed from the surface of the eye. The epithelium takes three or four days to heal. During this time you will experience discomfort and very blurry vision. By four or five days after surgery your vision begins to clear up, although it may takes several weeks to a month to become excellent. Visual clarity and crispness after PRK continue to improve for three to six months and then stabilize.

What happens if my vision isn't clear enough after PRK?

Even in the hands of a skilled surgeon, each person's eyes respond differently to the excimer laser, both during the surgery and while healing. Not everyone gets perfect vision. About 5 percent of PRK patients find their vision isn't as clear as they hoped. In this situation we usually recommend an enhancement procedure, which means doing another PRK procedure for the small residual correction. If you do need an enhancement procedure, it is usually done six months after the original surgery. An enhancement procedure can be performed years later if your eyesight changes over time.

How long will the correction last?

The results of your PRK do not diminish over time. Once your eyes have stabilized, usually in three to six months, your vision correction is permanent. This doesn't mean, however, that your vision won't change. Reading vision normally declines with age, and PRK doesn't prevent that decline. Also, vision is a combination of different parts of the eye, not just the cornea. Changes in other parts of the eye, like development of an early cataract, can change your vision. Usually, though, we find that vision stays excellent for many years to decades after PRK. If your vision does change when you are older, an enhancement procedure can usually be done to restore excellent vision without glasses.

Will I be able to drive immediately after PRK?

You can't drive the day of surgery because you will have blurry vision and may have taken a sedative. By the next morning, most people are seeing well enough to drive during the day without glasses. You should use good judgment, and drive only if you can see well enough to do so safely.

When can I go back to work?

Most patients can return to work four or five days after their PRK procedure.

If I have dry eyes, will it affect my PRK surgery?

That depends. Many people have PRK done because they have mild dry eyes and cannot wear contact lenses comfortably. These patients are delighted to have good vision without the irritation of contacts. On the other hand, if you have moderate or severe dry eyes, PRK may not be a good idea. Part of your comprehensive preoperative exam will be to evaluate your eyes for dryness and alert you if any abnormalities are found. Sometimes dry eyes can be treated preoperatively and you can still have successful PRK.

If I've had previous eye surgery, am I still a candidate for PRK?

Often, people who have had previous eye surgery are candidates for PRK. However, these can be more difficult surgeries and have less predictable results. For example, PRK has been used following an older form of refractive surgery, radial keratotomy (RK). With RK, the cornea is flattened by making small, spokelike incisions around its periphery to correct myopia and astigmatism. PRK following RK can succeed as long as the patient's vision is relatively stable and is still correctable with glasses.

If I have thin corneas, am I still a candidate for PRK?

Yes. PRK is the preferred procedure in patients with thin corneas because PRK does not sculpt as deeply into the cornea as LASIK.

Can I wear contact lenses after surgery, if needed?

After surgery, if you still need correction in one or both eyes, you may elect to wear contact lenses. Some patients who have monovision surgery will occasionally use a distance contact lens in the reading eye. They might do this in a situation where they want excellent distance vision in both eyes, such as playing tennis. If you tolerated the contacts before PRK, it is likely you will tolerate them afterward. In practice, though, rather than returning you to contact lens wear, your surgeon will generally recommend an enhancement to sharpen your vision.

Could the surgery cause problems years from now?

The chance of unknown complications years down the road is very unlikely. PRK is a form of lamellar refractive surgery, a type of surgery that has been performed since 1949. People who have undergone earlier types of lamellar refractive surgery—much less accurate and more invasive than PRK—have not developed unexpected problems during the past fifty years.

Will having PRK prevent eye diseases?

No. PRK does not prevent cataracts, glaucoma, retinal detachment, macular degeneration, or any other eye disease. That is why it is important to still have regular eye checkups after PRK, even if your vision is perfect. Equally true, PRK doesn't increase the risk of these problems or impair their treatment if you are diagnosed with these in the future.

Should I have both eyes done at the same time?

Some patients choose to have one eye treated at a time because of the relatively slow recovery from PRK. These patients rely on the unoperated on eye while the first eye recovers. Then, they get the second eye done. Most patients, however, prefer to do both eyes at once, to avoid going through the procedure twice and the recovery twice. In the end, the choice is yours, and you should feel no pressure to do it one way or the other.

Should I wait for the next generation of PRK treatment?

Recent years have brought several advancements to PRK surgery. We now routinely perform wavefront-guided PRK. This advanced way of measuring the eye prior to PRK surgery is described in detail in chapter 5 on LASIK. Wavefront-guided PRK gives a more accurate correction and better night vision than older forms of PRK.

Another advancement in PRK is the near-elimination of the risk of developing corneal haze after PRK. Better lasers and the use of an eyedrop called *mitomycin C* at the end of surgery nowadays results in crystal-clear corneas in almost everyone.

PRK is a fairly stable technology now, with advances happening incrementally. In general, people are getting older much faster than PRK is getting better. For most people, waiting longer doesn't make much sense; only incremental improvements are expected in the forseeable future.

7

Implantable Contact Lens

Many people want to get LASIK because their contacts are annoying or uncomfortable. They don't like having to take them in and out every night. They don't like losing them, tearing them, and having them fall out. Imagine how much happier people would be if they couldn't feel their contacts, never had to take them in and out, and didn't have to worry about packing lenses, cases, and solutions when they traveled. That dream can be a reality with the *implantable contact lens,* or *ICL* for short. Everyone has heard of LASIK, but the ICL is a better option for highly nearsighted individuals. More than a million ICLs have been implanted worldwide.

How the Implantable Contact Lens Corrects Your Vision

The ICL is a tiny contact lens, smaller than a dime, that is surgically inserted in your eye *(Figure 20)*. It floats in the space behind your iris and lens and you don't feel it *(Figure 21)*. It corrects your vision just like a regular contact lens, except you never have to clean it or remove it.

To implant the ICL, the surgeon makes a small incision, less than 1/8 inch wide, at the junction of the cornea and sclera (the white part of the eye). The lens is folded and gently inserted into the eye, where it unfurls. The lens is tucked behind the iris, and the procedure is over. No stitches are needed—the tiny incisions seal themselves.

Advantages of the ICL

The ICL is manufactured from a soft foldable material that contains natural collagen. Because the cornea is actually composed of collagen, this material provides excellent biocompatibility and superior optical capability.

The Implantable Contact Lens

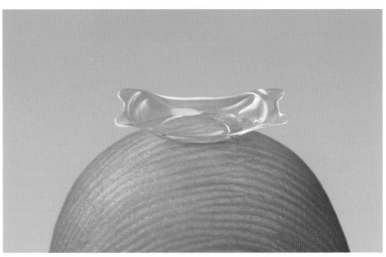

Figure 20. An implantable contact lens is soft and flexible, like a regular contact lens, but much smaller. The center portion of the lens corrects vision, and the four corners hold the lens in place in the eye.

Advantages of the ICL over LASIK or PRK include:

- *Quality of Vision*—Because the ICL can be manufactured to a high level of optical quality, it produces a crispness and clarity of vision that leaves many patients saying, "Wow, I've never seen this well."

- *Biocompatibility*—The collagen copolymer material of the ICL is not considered a foreign object by the body's immune system.

- *Comfort*—Patients can't feel the ICL in their eye.

- *Invisibility*—No one else can see the ICL in the eye.

- *Simplicity*—Unlike traditional contact lenses, once the ICL is implanted in the eye, there is no additional maintenance needed.

- *Removability*—The ICL is designed to be permanently placed in the eye. However, the lens can be removed if a patient's vision changes or if it needs to be removed or replaced for any reason.

Implanting the ICL

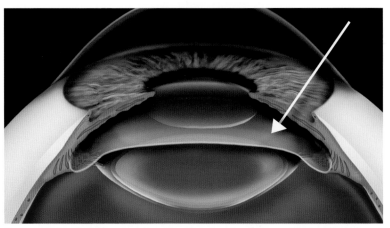

Figure 21. Soft and pliable, an implantable contact lens is rolled up and inserted into the eye through a tiny incision. It sits in front of the natural lens (*Arrow*). It provides excellent vision correction and is comfortable. It eliminates the routine removal and cleaning required of a regular contact lens.

The ICL and Astigmatism

The ICL can be made with astigmatism correction, just like soft contact lenses, so it can correct both nearsightedness and astigmatism

Are You a Candidate for the Implantable Contact Lens?

If you have a high level of nearsightedness, greater than –8.00 diopters, you are probably a strong candidate for the ICL. If you have a lower level of nearsightedness but you have corneas that are too thin for LASIK, the ICL may be an option for you. The ICL can correct your vision without the slow recovery you would have with PRK. The ICL doesn't make your eyes drier, so it can be a good option if you have significant dryness.

Some people aren't good candidates for the ICL. The ICL cannot correct farsightedness safely. Farsighted people have less room in the front part of their eyes, and there just isn't enough room to fit the lens. If you have a cataract, even a minor one, the ICL is not a good option. Refractive lens exchange (discussed in chapter 8) is a better option for people with cataracts.

Undergoing the ICL Procedure

The ICL procedure is somewhat more involved than LASIK, so most doctors, including us, have an anesthesiologist present to provide twilight anesthesia. This means you will get medications through an IV that make you very relaxed but not completely unconscious. This ensures you will be comfortable during the procedure.

Before the Procedure

A few days to a week before the ICL surgery, your doctor will have you come into the office to make a peripheral iridotomy. This is a tiny hole made with a laser at the edge of your iris (the colored part of the eye). The peripheral iridotomy allows fluid to circulate freely in the eye after the ICL is in place. The normal eye is filled with fluid that is made in the back part of the eye, behind the iris. The fluid flows through the pupil to the front part of the eye, where it drains out. The ICL is placed right behind the pupil so it can block this normal flow of fluid, which can allow pressure to build up in the back of the eye. The peripheral iridotomy allows fluid to flow normally to the front part of the eye, bypassing the pupil.

Making the peripheral iridotomy takes a couple of minutes per eye. You place your chin on a chin rest while the doctor operates the laser. You will feel mild momentary discomfort during the laser treatment, but there is no need for anesthesia, an IV, or sedation. You can drive home immediately afterward.

The Day of Your Procedure

There are some things you need to do to prepare for your surgery. It is important not to eat for six hours prior to the procedure, because it is possible that you would regurgitate food in your stomach while you are sedated, causing pneumonia. If you do eat or drink anything during this time, even a cup of coffee, your surgery will be canceled. You should, however, take your usual medications with small sips of water.

Make sure all makeup is cleaned off your eye and face before you come in. Don't wear jewelry or other valuables. Do wear comfortable street clothes—you'll be wearing them during surgery, so make sure they're loose-fitting, not binding. Bring a list of the medications you're taking to the surgery center; the anesthesiologist needs to be aware of all drugs you're currently taking. If you wear contact lenses, remove the lens from the eye to be treated twenty-four hours before surgery and leave it out.

Arrange for someone to drive you home after surgery. This is important because you will not be able to drive right after surgery; you'll be a little groggy from the sedative and your pupil will be dilated. Plan to spend about two and a half hours at the center.

How the Procedure Is Performed

In the preoperative area, the nurse starts an IV and dilates your pupil. A surgical cap is placed over your hair. Your pupils are dilated for thirty to forty-five minutes. You are taken to the operating room, where you are positioned lying comfortably on a surgical bed. The anesthesiologist gives you sedation through your IV. You are given eyedrops to numb the eyes, which may sting for a few seconds. Your face is cleaned with a disinfectant. More numbing eyedrops are given.

The surgeon then does the procedure. First a small incision is made in the edge of your cornea, just next to the white part of the eye (the sclera). The soft, flexible ICL is rolled up into a long cylinder and inserted through the incision. It unfolds in the eye. The surgeon tucks the ICL behind the pupil, in front of the natural lens. No stitches are needed because the tiny incision seals itself. The entire procedure takes about seven minutes. You are sedated the whole time, so you aren't nervous and don't feel pain.

After the procedure, your vision is hazy because your eye is still dilated, but you immediately notice that you can see much better. You can read a clock across the room. Once the sedation has worn off, in about twenty minutes, you can go home. You will be sent home with antibiotic and anti-inflammatory drops to promote healing. With the ICL procedure, one eye is done at a time, with the second eye scheduled one week later.

Recovering from the Procedure

The day after surgery is very exciting. Most likely you will be seeing 20/20 or better. Usually, you will drive yourself to the checkup the day after surgery without glasses. For someone who has been severely nearsighted his or her entire adult life, the effect is miraculous. You can't feel the lens and your eyes are comfortable.

The main concern for the first few days after surgery is making sure that your eye pressure stays normal. On rare occasions the peripheral iridotomy gets plugged up and the fluid can't circulate normally so pressure builds up in your eye. The pressure causes an aching feeling in your eye, your temple, or your cheek. If this happens, the surgeon will likely do more laser treatment to enlarge the peripheral iridotomy, which ensures the pressure stays normal. The most important thing to note is this: if you feel pressure or a headachy feeling in or around your eye, call the surgeon immediately, even if it is the middle of the night. Don't wait and hope it will go away.

Postoperative Care

You will typically see your ophthalmologist the day after your procedure for a checkup, and again during the first week after the procedure. You will use eyedrops containing a steroid to promote healing. Keeping your follow-up appointments is important, even if your vision is perfect. Your doctor needs to monitor your healing to be sure it is normal.

Resuming Activities

Don't drive on the day of surgery. Resume driving only when your vision is clear enough that you are safe on the road, which is usually the next morning for most people. Also, stay away from swimming pools, Jacuzzis, and hot tubs for a week after surgery. Bacteria in the water could cause an infection. It is fine to shower or bathe, though, because tap water has very few bacteria.

It is fine to wear makeup, but avoid wearing old mascara and eyeliner for the first week after the procedure. Old mascara and eyeliner can accumulate germs, which you do not want to introduce into your eyes. If you wish to wear mascara or eyeliner during the first week after surgery, open a fresh tube. For the same reason, avoid dusty environments for the first three days.

Otherwise, there are very few restrictions on your activities after your surgery. Reading, computer work, watching television, and flying are all fine to do immediately. You can restart your regular exercise regimen the morning after surgery.

Results You Can Expect from the ICL

The U.S. Armed Forces have been enthusiastic adopters of the ICL because it offers the excellent night vision critical to soldiers in combat. In one large study done by the U.S. military, 98 percent of patients achieved 20/20 vision or better with the ICL and 80 percent could see 20/15. Even though not everyone saw 20/20, 99 percent of patients said they were satisfied with the results. These superb results may overstate the accuracy of the ICL somewhat because many of the patients in the study were not extreme myopes. Nevertheless, the excellent visual results in this study well illustrate the effectiveness of the ICL.

If you aren't 20/20 after the ICL surgery, you can have a LASIK touch-up to improve your vision further. LASIK touch-ups are typically done three months after the ICL procedure, to give your eye time to heal fully. If you are in a hurry, a PRK touch-up can be done as soon as a month after ICL surgery, but the recovery from LASIK is so much faster that patients typically wait for LASIK.

If you are forty-two years old or older, you will need reading glasses after the ICL surgery because you will have excellent distance vision but will have difficulty reading because of presbyopia. If you are over age forty, we will often do monovision to give you excellent close-up vision. Monovision works well after the ICL surgery, just as it does after PRK or LASIK.

Potential Complications with the ICL Surgery

The ICL has some definite safety advantages over other procedures. It is removable, unlike other procedures. It doesn't make the eyes drier. It usually offers better night vision than LASIK or PRK. It also offers sharper quality of vision than these two procedures. Just as all surgical procedures carry risks, so does the ICL procedure. However, when ICL surgery is performed by an experienced surgeon, the risk of complications is quite low.

We've listed both the rare and serious complications and the less rare and mild ones. Although this list is not exhaustive, it includes the complications that you need to know about in order to be comfortable about proceeding with surgery.

Undercorrection

Undercorrection means that your nearsightedness wasn't fully corrected by the ICL, so you are still a little bit nearsighted. A slight undercorrection will not seriously affect your vision and is often desirable in patients over forty to help with their reading vision. If the undercorrection is enough to cause significant blurring of vision, your surgeon will recommend an enhancement procedure for you.

Overcorrection

Overcorrection means that your nearsightedness was corrected more than intended, leaving you farsighted. Far-sightedness can make it harder to see clearly up close. As with undercorrections, a significant overcorrection can be treated with an enhancement procedure.

The most common enhancement procedure done after ICL surgery is LASIK, and it is usually performed three months after the ICL procedure. LASIK can easily correct small amounts of residual nearsightedness, farsightedness, or astigmatism. If LASIK is a good enhancement procedure for patients after ICL surgery, you may wonder why the surgeon doesn't do LASIK in the first place. The reason is that LASIK is good for small or moderate corrections, but not good for the high corrections where the ICL shines.

Presbyopia

Loss of close vision is a natural part of aging. As discussed earlier, we call this process presbyopia. Presbyopia occurs slightly sooner with the ICL. Normally, people with excellent vision get reading glasses at age forty-five. If you are corrected for excellent distance vision with the ICL, you will probably need reading glasses at the age of forty-two or forty-three. This happens for optical reasons that are beyond the scope of this book. If you are over the age of forty, monovision with the ICL may be an excellent option for you.

Nighttime Halos and Starburst

As described earlier in this book, halos occur when you are in a dark environment and look at a small bright light, such as a headlight or a streetlight. Halo is the glow that surrounds the light. Starburst is little spiky rays of light that emanate from the light source. Everyone has some degree of halos and starburst at night, even if they haven't had refractive surgery. Look carefully at a headlight or streetlight tonight so you understand what we're talking about.

The ICL generally offers better night vision than LASIK. However, the ICL can still cause an increase in halos and starburst around lights at night. When the pupil dilates at night, it is larger than the diameter of the ICL. The light that enters the eye through the pupil outside the edge of the ICL will cause halos. These symptoms can be bothersome in dim light conditions, such as driving at night. Our experience is that patients like great vision much more than they are bothered by the halos. On the occasions that patients have mentioned that they have more halos after surgery, we have offered to remove the ICL to restore their night vision to its preoperative state. Not once has a patient taken us up on the offer. What we hear instead is, "No way! I don't want my vision to go back to the way it was."

As described earlier, the peripheral iridotomy is a tiny hole that is made to allow fluid to flow from the back of the eye to the front of the eye. A small amount of light can pass through this hole and create starburst, particularly at night. For this reason, the hole is intentionally made very small, to minimize the amount of light that enters, and is placed, if possible, under the upper eyelid, so that the eyelid blocks the entrance of light.

Increased Eye Pressure

A rare complication of the ICL is a sudden rise in eye pressure. This may happen in the first week after surgery when fluid can't flow from the back of the eye to the front through the iridotomy. If this happens you will feel a strong aching pain in your eyeball or in the area around the eye. It feels like a sinus headache. You may also experience nausea. If you have an aching pain or nausea in the first week after surgery, it is important to contact your doctor, even if it is the middle of the night. The doctor will be able to relieve the pain very quickly. Don't wait, because it will just get worse.

A sudden rise in eye pressure can occur in two situations. The first situation is if the iridotomy is not big enough. Fluid can't flow through it, and the pressure rises. This is easily treated by enlarging the iridotomy with the laser in the doctor's office. The second situation is if the ICL is too big for your eye. The ICL comes in different sizes. We measure your eye carefully prior to surgery to determine the correct size, but it is not an exact science. On rare occasions the ICL is too big. In this case the overlarge ICL pushes on the peripheral iridotomy and closes it. This situation is treated by removing the ICL and replacing it with a smaller lens.

Cataract

Cataract is a haziness that develops in the natural crystalline lens of the eye. It is a natural part of aging, like gray hair. Everyone gets a cataract if they live long enough. Highly nearsighted people—those who are candidates for ICL surgery—often get cataracts in their sixties or seventies. Cataracts are easy to treat with cataract surgery. In this operation, the hazy natural lens is removed and replaced with a clear synthetic lens.

The ICL slightly increases your chance of getting a cataract earlier in life, but the chance is small. In the FDA study of the ICL, approximately 1 percent of eyes with the ICL needed cataract surgery each year. If you develop a cataract after your ICL surgery, the ICL is removed as the first step in the cataract surgery, and the new synthetic lens is chosen so your nearsightedness is still corrected after the cataract surgery.

Rare Complications

Infection inside the eye can occur after ICL surgery, but is extremely rare. It is a feared complication because an infection inside the eye can damage vital tissues. None of the 526 eyes that had surgery in the large FDA study of the ICL developed an eye infection. Careful surgeons use a technique that minimizes the risk of infection. This involves doing the ICL procedure under very sterile conditions, sterilizing the eye carefully before surgery, and using antibiotics in the eye at the end of surgery to prevent infection.

If your eye does become infected, it will likely occur during the first forty-eight to seventy-two hours after the ICL surgery. This is why it is important for the first week after surgery to avoid any contact with substances that carry bacteria, such as old eye makeup, hot tubs, and swimming pools. It is also essential to go to all of your follow-up visits, even if everything seems fine.

Any eye surgery can result in loss of vision. Fortunately, this is extremely rare with ICL. Our practice has never had a patient lose his or her vision from ICL surgery, and no patients in the large FDA study lost vision from the ICL.

Frequently Asked Questions about ICL Surgery

Your doctor should take the time to answer any questions you may have. Here are the most common questions we hear regarding ICL surgery.

Can other people see the ICL in my eye?

No. The placement of the ICL behind the iris makes the lens invisible to you and anyone else, even if they look closely.

Can I feel the ICL in my eye?

No. Unlike a regular contact lenses, which cause dryness and irritation, the ICL can't be felt in your eye.

What if my vision changes?

The ICL may be removed or replaced if your eyesight changes, but normally we would do a simple LASIK enhancement to "tune up" your vision if it changes.

Does the lens ever wear out or need replacement?

No. The lens never wears out.

Can the lenses get dirty like a contact lens?

No. The ICL will always remain clear. It is maintenance free.

Can I open my eyes under water?

Yes. Because the lens is inside your eye, it isn't affected by water, rain, or steam.

Why haven't I heard of the ICL?

These days, most people still have LASIK. In our practice, we recommend the ICL to about 5 percent of people who come to us for consultation. That means that, on average, you would need to know twenty people who have had refractive surgery to know one person who has had the ICL. Still, more than 375,000 ICL implants have been done around the world.

Why is the ICL procedure popular in the U.S. military services?

The U.S. military loves the ICL for two reasons. First, the recovery is quick, so soldiers are back on duty quickly. Second, the clarity of vision is outstanding. For a combat soldier, perhaps more than for any other profession, clear vision is vital. Clear vision can truly mean the difference between life and death.

8

Refractive Lens Exchange

The natural lens in your eye is an important contributor to your eye's ability to focus light. In fact, your natural lens having the wrong power is a common cause of nearsightedness and farsightedness. As discussed in previous chapters, LASIK and PRK correct nearsightedness and farsightedness by changing the focusing power of the cornea. Another way to correct nearsightedness or farsightedness is to change the focusing power of the lens. We do this by removing the lens and replacing it with a new lens with the correct power to give you good vision. This operation is called *refractive lens exchange* or *RLE* for short.

Both refractive lens exchange and the ICL procedure involve inserting a synthetic lens in your eye, but they are different procedures. In RLE, the natural lens is removed, while in the ICL procedure it is left in place.

How Refractive Lens Exchange Corrects Your Vision

The surgeon makes a small incision and inserts a thin vibrating probe to gently vacuum your natural lens out of the eye. A new synthetic lens is implanted to correct your vision. This synthetic lens is called an *intraocular lens implant,* or *IOL (Figure 22)*. The lens implant is folded and inserted through the incision, and then unfolded and positioned in the eye. The incision is so small that it seals itself, so no sutures are needed. The entire procedure is painless and generally takes about ten minutes per eye.

If you are farsighted, your natural lens is not strong enough. The surgeon removes your natural lens and inserts a lens implant of stronger power to correct your farsightedness.

The Intraocular Lens (IOL)

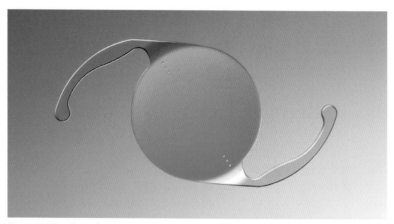

Figure 22. The photo above shows an intraocular lens (IOL), the synthetic lens that is inserted during a refractive lens exchange surgery. The two "arms" on each side of the lens hold it in place. *Photo courtesy of Alcon Inc.*

Similarly, if you are nearsighted, the surgeon removes your natural lens and inserts a weaker lens implant.

Recovery is rapid—you can resume most of your normal activities the next day. Within a day or two of your surgery, you'll marvel at how clear and vivid your world has become without glasses. In the hands of an experienced eye surgeon, refractive lens exchange is among the most effective and safe surgical procedures.

Choices in Lens Implants

Modern intraocular lenses are made of polymer materials that have proven to be very well tolerated in the eye over decades of use. They are flexible so they can be rolled up to fit through a very small incision. Once inside the eye, they unfold to about a quarter of an inch in size. Side struts, called haptics, hold them in place inside the eye. The lens implants become part of the eye. They are safe, stable, and reliable, and they require no care or maintenance other than general practices for good eye health *(Figure 23).*

A variety of lens implants are available that have different capabilities. Your doctor will recommend the particular type of lens whose capabilities most match your needs. In general terms, there are currently three different types of lens implants

IOL Placement

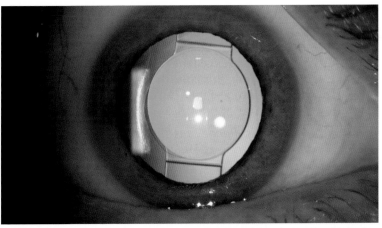

Figure 23. Photo of another type of intraocular lens implant (IOL) in the eye. In refractive lens exchange (RLE), the natural lens is removed from the eye through a tiny incision and replaced with an IOL. The power of the IOL is chosen to correct nearsightedness, farsightedness, and astigmatism.

that can replace your natural lens, and a fourth type that will be here soon. The four types are:

- monofocal or standard lens
- toric lens
- multifocal and extended range lenses
- light-adjustable lenses

Monofocal or Standard Lens Implant

The *monofocal lens implant,* also called the *standard lens implant,* has a single fixed focal point. This lens provide precise vision at a particular distance. With refractive lens exchange, the lens implant in one eye is usually set for excellent distance vision. The other eye may also be set for excellent distance vision, or it may be set for reading or intermediate vision, to create monovision. (*See* chapter 2 for a detailed discussion of monovision). The monofocal lens is ideal for those who want very crisp vision.

Toric Lens Implant

The *toric lens implant* is a single-focus lens implant that also has a built-in ability to correct astigmatism. Astigmatism means that your cornea is oval-shaped like a football instead of round like a basketball. If you have significant astigmatism and it isn't corrected, your vision won't be perfectly clear at any distance. The toric lens implant is an excellent way to correct astigmatism and provide very crisp vision at the chosen distance. Monovision can also be done with the toric lens implant to provide both excellent reading and distance vision. Like the monofocal lens implant, the toric lens provides very crisp vision. If you have a significant astigmatism, the toric lens is the best lens implant option for you.

Multifocal and Extended-Range Lens Implants

The *multifocal* and *extended-range lens implants* have different focusing zones built into the lens, allowing a wide range of vision with decreased dependence on glasses *(Figure 24)*. The multifocal lens implant provides good distance and reading vision, and the extended-range lens implant provides good distance and intermediate vision. Unlike standard spectacle bifocal lenses, you don't have to look up to see far away and look down to read. You can see close and far in any direction you look. These lens implants work by dividing the light that enters the eye, focusing half the light for distance vision and the other half for close or intermediate vision.

Because of the way they focus light, these lenses have two disadvantages. They produce five or six concentric circles, called halos, around headlights and streetlights at night. These halos can be bothersome during night driving. The other disadvantage is that distance vision is not as sharp as it is with monofocal and toric implants, because part of the incoming light is being used for close vision. Your doctor will discuss with you whether a multifocal or extended-range lens implant would be appropriate for you.

Light-Adjustable lens

We are particularly excited about a newer lens implant, the *light-adjustable lens* or *LAL* for short. The light-adjustable lens is a remarkable lens implant whose power can be adjusted after surgery by shining an ultraviolet light on the lens. Sometimes after refractive lens exchange (or any of our procedures), patients find their vision is much better but not quite perfect because of mild residual nearsightedness, farsightedness, or astigmatism. When this happens with other lens implants, we

Multifocal IOL

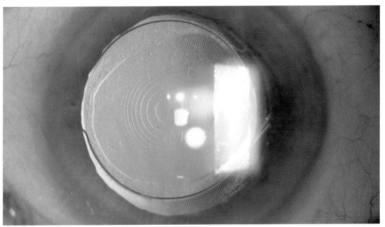

Figure 24. A multifocal IOL has a series of concentric rings etched on the lens that provide both a far and close focus. This allows good distance and reading vision without glasses.

do a LASIK enhancement. With the light-adjustable lens, by precisely controlling the pattern of light, the lens implant itself can be adjusted to correct any remaining refractive error after RLE surgery. The result is extraordinarily clear vision.

The light-adjustable lens does require a greater commitment from you. Since ultraviolet light changes the lens power, you need to wear sunglasses outdoors for the first few weeks after surgery. It also requires extra visits to the doctor, because the adjustment of the lens power is done in one or two steps, followed by a "lock-in" step that freezes the power of the lens permanently, so it is no longer affected by sunlight. We see the light adjustable lens as a twenty-second century technology that arrived a century early.

The variety of lens implants available makes refractive lens exchange a very flexible and customizable approach to optimizing your vision without glasses.

Refractive Lens Exchange: Sister Operation to Cataract Surgery

For a moment, allow us to digress and mention cataracts and cataract surgery. As we age, many tissues in our bodies begin to deteriorate. Our hair goes gray and our backs ache.

Cataract

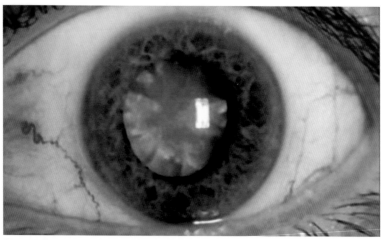

Figure 25. A cataract is a clouding of the natural lens of the eye. It makes vision blurry and is treated by replacing the cloudy lens with an intraocular lens.

The lenses in our eyes also deteriorate. The deterioration of the lens first shows up in our forties as presbyopia. Then, sometime after we turn sixty, we start to develop cataracts. A cataract is haziness in the natural lens of the eye *(Figure 25)*. It causes hazy vision, like looking through waxed paper or a very dirty windshield.

Everyone gets a cataract eventually, if they live long enough; it is as certain as gray hair. Nowadays, cataracts are easily treated with cataract surgery. In cataract surgery, the hazy natural lens of the eye is removed and replaced with a clear lens.

Why the digression about cataract surgery in a chapter on refractive lens exchange? Because cataracts involve the same operation performed for refractive lens exchange. No doubt you know someone who has had cataract surgery—it is the most common surgical procedure performed in the United States, with more than 3 million procedures performed annually. Refractive lens exchange is simply cataract surgery performed on an eye where there is no cataract. In fact, one of the great advantages of RLE is that it uses the same advanced technology and proven techniques that have been used for years in cataract surgery.

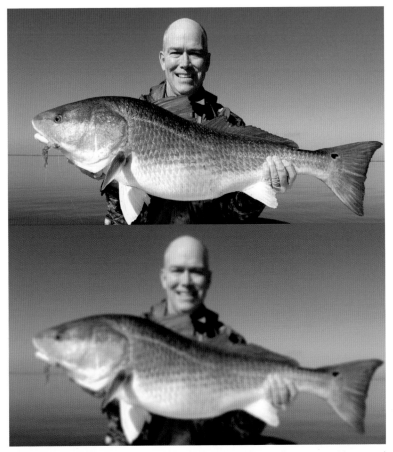

Author, Dr. Robert K. Maloney, with a big fish! The top photo shows colors as seen with a normal eye. The photo on the bottom shows colors as they may appear with a cataract.

A significant advantage of RLE is that you can never get a cataract because your natural lens has been replaced by a synthetic lens that will never get hazy. You will never need to have cataract surgery in the future. That's nice because that's one aging problem taken care of that you won't have to worry about later, when perhaps you aren't as healthy. With refractive lens exchange, you are basically killing two birds with one stone—eliminating the need for glasses now and the need for cataract surgery later.

Many farsighted people in their fifties and sixties choose to have refractive lens exchange before cataracts have a chance to develop. These people don't want to wear eyeglasses or contacts, and they choose not to have other forms of refractive surgery, such as LASIK, because within a few years they might well need cataract surgery anyway. With RLE, just as with cataract surgery, your surgeon will explain the choices you have in choosing an intraocular lens.

Are You a Candidate for RLE?

Two conditions make you an optimal candidate for RLE. The first is if you have moderate to severe farsightedness. LASIK isn't very good at correcting higher levels of farsightedness because the effect tends to partially wear off over time, so you may have to go back to wearing glasses. Also, the crispness of vision isn't as good when higher levels of farsightedness are corrected with LASIK. For this condition, RLE offers crisper vision than LASIK and a permanent correction.

The other condition that makes you a strong candidate for refractive lens exchange is having the beginning of a cataract in your eye. Even if the cataract is not yet affecting your vision, it makes more sense to have RLE rather than some other procedure, such as LASIK, and then need to undergo cataract surgery in the near future. Also, the other vision correction procedures often don't work as well if there is a beginning cataract.

Undergoing the RLE Procedure

Your eye surgeon will give you specific instructions to follow before and after your procedure and will tell you what to expect during the procedure. The routine can vary from clinic to clinic and from doctor to doctor. If what you read in the following paragraphs differs from your doctor's instructions, follow your doctor's instructions instead.

Before the Procedure

There are some things you need to do to prepare for your surgery. It is important not to eat for six hours prior to the procedure. If you do eat or drink anything during this time, even a cup of coffee, your surgery will be canceled. You should, however, take your usual medications with small sips of water.

Light Adjustable Lens

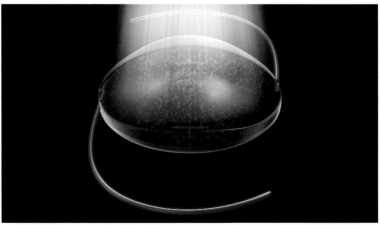

Light adjustable lenses are made of silicone that can be shaped by ultraviolet light after the lens is placed in the eye. This process allows for the correction of any remaining nearsightedness, farsightedness, and astigmatism after cataract surgery.

Make sure all makeup is cleaned off your eye and face before you come in. Don't wear jewelry or other valuables. Do wear comfortable street clothes. These are the clothes you'll be wearing during surgery, so make sure they're loose-fitting and comfortable. Bring of list of your medications to the surgery center—the anesthesiologist needs to be aware of any drugs you're currently taking. If you wear contact lenses, remove the lens from the eye to be treated twenty-four hours before surgery and leave it out.

Arrange for someone to drive you home after surgery. This is important because you will not be able to drive right after surgery: you'll be a little groggy from the sedative and your pupil will be dilated. Plan to spend about two and a half hours at the center.

How the Procedure Is Performed

About forty-five minutes before the surgery, a nurse will put drops in your eye to dilate your pupil. In the operating room, your eyelid, eyelashes, and face will be cleaned with an antibacterial iodine solution. This minimizes any possibility of infection. The iodine cleansing is one of several ways of ensuring that the procedure is completely sterile.

The anesthesiologist will give you a strong sedative through an IV line. The sedative won't put you completely to sleep, but you will be sleepy and relaxed during surgery.

You'll lie on your back, covered with a special sterile sheet that has an opening over the eye. The rest of your face will be covered to keep bacteria from your nose and mouth away from your eye. While your face is covered, a tube releases a flow of oxygen toward your face so you can breathe comfortably. The anesthesiologist will be sitting by your side the entire time, monitoring your vital signs throughout the procedure and giving you more sedation if you feel anxious.

The actual refractive lens exchange procedure takes about ten minutes per eye and is painless. The surgeon numbs your eye, then makes a tiny incision at the edge of the cornea. No needles are used. The surgeon inserts a thin vibrating probe through the incision to break up your natural lens and vacuum out the fragments. He or she will leave in place the membrane that surrounds the natural lens. This membrane is called the *capsular bag*. The capsular bag supports the new intraocular lens implant. The lens implant is inserted and positioned. The incision is self-sealing because it is so small; no sutures are needed. You will return to the recovery room, where a nurse will check your blood pressure again, give you something to eat or drink, and monitor you for a half hour. Then you can go home.

Recovering from the RLE Procedure

Your pupil is dilated and will stay dilated overnight, so you will notice that your vision is blurry and you will feel light-sensitive until the next day. Your eye should be comfortable after surgery, although you will notice a scratchy feeling on the day of surgery. It is fine to take your preferred pain reliever for this. You should have no more than a mild aching feeling in or around your eye. If there is more than minor pain, you should notify your surgeon. Feel free to watch television or go out to dinner with friends. There should be no redness or puffiness, and you will be able to see well enough to get around.

Your doctor will probably operate on one eye at a time, typically doing the procedures two weeks apart. This way the doctor can make sure that the first eye is healing properly before doing the second eye.

Postoperative Care

You will come into the office the day after your procedure for a checkup, and again during the first week. You will use several different eyedrops. These include a steroid drop to promote healing and a liquid version of aspirin that reduces inflammation. Keeping your follow-up appointments is important, even if your vision is perfect. Your doctor needs to monitor your healing to be sure it is normal.

Resuming Activities

Don't drive on the day of surgery. Resume driving only when your vision is clear enough that you are safe on the road, which is the next morning for most people. Also, stay away from swimming pools, Jacuzzis, and hot tubs for a week after surgery. Bacteria in the water could cause an infection. It is fine to shower or bathe, though, because tap water has very few bacteria.

It is fine to wear makeup, but avoid wearing old mascara and eyeliner for the first week. Old mascara and eyeliner can accumulate germs, which you do not want to introduce into your eyes. If you wish to wear mascara or eyeliner during the first week after surgery, open a fresh tube. For the same reason, avoid dusty environments for the first three days.

Otherwise, there are very few restrictions on your activities after your surgery. Reading, computer work, watching television, and flying are all fine to do immediately. You may exercise the morning after surgery. You may require a thin pair of glasses for reading. A pair of magnifiers from the drugstore should work fine.

Results You Can Expect from RLE

You'll be able to enjoy greater independence and a wider range of activities after RLE surgery. And all this will be possible with less dependence—maybe even no dependence—on eyeglasses. Your world will be brighter and clearer. You'll be able to focus better. Typically, you'll see well enough to watch television and go out to dinner immediately after surgery, and drive a car and exercise the next day, all without glasses. If you had a monovision correction or a multifocal lens implant, you will typically be able to read a menu, a newspaper, and your cell phone without glasses. Statistically, about 75 percent of patients achieve 20/25 or better vision after the RLE procedure. If your vision is not good enough, LASIK enhancement can be done to refine it.

No replacement lens, however sophisticated it might be, is as good as a young, healthy, crystal-clear natural lens. Though your vision will almost certainly be better than before your surgery, it will not be as sharp as a teenager's. You may find that although your distance vision is good enough to see almost everything far away, you may still put on a pair of glasses for night driving or other situations in which you need perfect vision. Also, refractive lens exchange isn't the fountain of youth. Even with monovision or a multifocal lens implant, you still probably won't be able to read the tiny print on a label without some reading glasses, but you will be much less dependent on glasses.

Your vision will fluctuate for a week or longer, depending on the type of lens implanted. Even so, within twenty-four hours your eyesight will be markedly improved—so much so that you'll probably be eager to schedule surgery for the other eye as soon as possible.

Potential Complications with RLE

Refractive lens exchange is a safe procedure, and complications are rare. Still, you should be aware of possible side effects and potential problems, which are discussed following.

Residual Nearsightedness or Farsightedness

As with other refractive surgeries, we can't be sure you'll achieve exactly the vision that was planned. We do detailed measurements of your eye prior to surgery to achieve the most accurate possible result, but each person responds to the surgery differently and heals slightly differently. Even if your vision isn't perfect, it should still be very good. If the imperfection is bothersome or disappointing, a LASIK enhancement surgery can be done to correct the small residual refractive error. Normally, we wait three months before doing the LASIK touch-up to let your eye heal fully.

If you have received the light-adjustable lens, of course, this isn't a problem. The doctor simply shines a special pattern of ultraviolet light on your eye to correct your vision, without the need for a LASIK enhancement.

Starburst or Halos

Everyone, whether or not they have had RLE, experiences some starburst or halos at night. These night-vision disturbances occur when you are in a dark environment and look at a small bright light, such as a headlight or a streetlight. Halo is the glow that surrounds the light source, and starburst is little spiky rays of light that emanate from the light source. Look carefully at a headlight or streetlight tonight so you understand what we're talking about.

You may notice more starburst and halos after RLE. These symptoms usually are not bothersome, but some find them annoying in dim light conditions, such as driving at night. If you elected to have a multifocal lens implant, you will typically notice four or five small halos around lights at night.

If you develop more starburst or halos after RLE, there are treatment options. Glasses with a light prescription for night driving can help, as can the use at dusk of eyedrops that reduce the size of your pupils.

Shadow from the Edge of the Lens Implant

It is possible for light coming from your far peripheral vision to pass through the pupil and reflect off the edge of the lens implant. When this happens, you will typically see a light or dark arc in your far peripheral vision. This is called a *dysphotopsia*. It can be annoying because it looks as if something is getting in the way of your peripheral vision. It will not affect your central vision or your clarity of vision. It is similar to seeing the frame around a pair of eyeglasses, but less bothersome because it is more peripheral. These disappear in most people during the first year after surgery.

Posterior Capsule Opacification

When the natural lens is removed, the membrane that surrounds the natural lens, the capsular bag, is left in place to hold the new lens implant. The back part of this membrane is called the *posterior capsule*. Sometimes, the posterior capsule becomes cloudy after surgery, caused by the body's natural healing response. This cloudiness—which can develop months or years after your surgery—is called *posterior capsule opacification*. It is quite common and affects younger patients more often than older patients.

Posterior capsule opacification can be quickly and safely corrected with a three-minute outpatient procedure called *YAG laser capsulotomy*. Your eye surgeon will use a laser beam to make a small opening in the back of the posterior capsule, allowing light through. The procedure is painless and requires no incision or sutures.

Floaters

You'll see everything more clearly—including *floaters,* those little objects that drift across your field of vision. If you notice something that looks like a few gnats or strands flying across your field of vision when you move your eyes, it's nothing to be concerned about. If the floaters are bothersome, there are treatments for these—either a laser treatment to break up the floaters or a surgery to remove them entirely.

Retinal Detachment

Retinal detachment is a separation of the retina from the inner wall of the eye. This is very rare in farsighted eyes, but less rare in highly nearsighted eyes (which is why we prefer to do RLE in farsighted eyes). It is treated with another operation, called *retinal reattachment surgery.* Symptoms of retinal detachment include a shower of new floaters, much like a swarm of bees, in your vision, or repetitive flashes, like fireworks, of light in your peripheral vision. The most distinctive symptom is a dark curtain moving across your vision in the affected eye; the dark area is the region of the retina that has already detached If you have these symptoms after RLE, notify your doctor immediately.

Other Possible Complications

There are some possible but rare complications from RLE. In perhaps 0.5 percent of eyes, a break in the posterior capsule can occur during surgery. When this happens, it may be necessary to use a lens implant different from the one you chose before surgery. Infection can occur, in fewer than one-tenth of 1 percent of patients. This is treated with an operation, called a *vitrectomy,* to remove the infection and inject antibiotics into the eye. Accumulation of fluid in the macula can cause blurry vision and can usually be managed using anti-inflammatory eyedrops. Swelling of the cornea can also cause blurred vision. Rarely, the lens implant shifts or rotates within the eye. If this occurs, it can be repositioned surgically, although wearing thin eyeglasses usually solves the problem. Although it is possible to lose your vision in the eye from RLE or any operation, these rare complications can usually be treated successfully if caught in time.

Frequently Asked Questions about RLE

Is the RLE procedure painful?

No. Using numbing eyedrops and intravenous sedation, we keep you very comfortable.

Having someone perform surgery on my eye makes me anxious. Should I be nervous?

Being nervous is understandable. But the IV sedation takes away the feeling of anxiety. Afterward, you'll be amazed at how easily the surgery went.

Can I see the surgery being performed?

Not really. You will see bright lights and kaleidoscopic colors, like a light show, but you can't see surgical instruments and surgical maneuvers. Because of the sedation, you aren't aware of much.

Will I be able to feel the lens implant in my eye?

No. The lens becomes a natural part of your body.

Can other people see the lens implant in my eye?

No. The lens is not visible. However, when the light is just right, others may see a faint reflection off the surface of the lens right in the center of your pupil, almost like a gleam in your eye.

Does the lens need to be replaced eventually?

No. The lens is made of extremely durable polymers that have been implanted safely in people for decades. The lens will outlast you.

9

Choosing an Eye Surgeon

If you have gotten this far in the book, you understand why you need glasses, what vision correction procedure you may be qualified for, and what the advantages and disadvantages are of that procedure. Now you must choose an experienced eye surgeon. It's difficult because you are on the outside looking in, trying to make sense of a surgeon's abilities and qualifications. In this chapter, we'll help you peek under the hood so you can recognize the best surgeons amid the average ones.

Selecting the best surgeon is important. Vision correction surgery is remarkably safe, but it is still surgery—surgery on your eyes, your most important connection to the outside world. It is worth your time and effort to determine which doctor will get you the best result because you'll live with that result for the rest of your life. You should evaluate a potential surgeon in three major categories: reputation, credentials, and practice style.

Surgeon's Reputation

We think reputation is the best indicator of quality because reputations can't be bought. They can only be earned, and only earned by doing great work for a long time on a lot of patients. Pay close attention to reputation in choosing your surgeon. There are several ways to get a read on a surgeon's reputation.

Ask Other Patients

If you know people who have had vision correction surgery, ask them who their surgeon was and how they felt about their overall experience. Were they happy with the outcome? Did they have confidence in their surgeon? Was the surgeon compassionate, and did he or she take time to answer questions before and after the procedure? Was the care personalized or did the office feel like a too-busy bus station? Personal experiences are powerful indicators of the quality of care. Don't rely on a single patient referral, though. Ask lots of people to get a more complete picture.

Ask Your Optometrist

Eye doctors know who the best surgeons are, and they are usually better able than you are to assess a surgeon's talents. An eye care practitioner whom you trust and respect is a great source of referrals. Because referring patients is a routine and important part of their professional practice, these physicians will almost always be able to recommend a nearby surgeon with a sound reputation. They can't afford to refer to a bad provider because patients hold them responsible if they make a bad referral.

Ask Other Eye Doctors

Call other local eye doctors' offices and ask whom they refer patients for LASIK, or whichever surgery you are considering. Many doctors will provide this information over the phone without a need to visit. Even smarter is to call other LASIK surgeons outside your state (find them on the Internet). Tell whoever answers the phone that you heard their doctor is great but it is too far for you to travel. Ask if they would recommend a surgeon in your area. A little flattery will likely get you the names of surgeons in your area who have a reputation that has spread nationwide. These are the surgeons who should do your surgery. Nobody knows the abilities and limitations of a surgeon better than other surgeons who do the same thing.

Search the Internet

If you do research on the Internet, you will find much information about vision correction surgery. Online review sites are a good place to learn about a doctor's practice style. Read both the good and bad reviews. Even the best surgeons will have some bad reviews, but bad reviews should be a low percentage. Read the bad reviews and see how the doctor responds (if at all). Is the doctor's response caring and conciliatory, or hostile and defensive? You'll learn how he or she handles unhappy patients. There are review sites specifically dedicated to reviewing professionals, but at this time they aren't getting the traction that Yelp and Google have.

Check Doctor Ratings

Two organizations identify the best doctors in each geographic area and specialty. These organizations survey a large number of doctors and ask the question, "If you or a member of your family had a medical problem, who would you turn to for help?" The better organization is *America's Top Doctors,* which has an excellent website that allows you to search for doctors in your area (www.castleconnolly.com). Only the best 1 percent or 2 percent of doctors make this listing. The other organization is *Best Doctors in America.* It identifies the top 5 percent of American physicians. Its website is not searchable, but the doctors chosen by this organization will often have a recognition plaque in their office. Being listed by either of these organizations is a strong sign that the surgeon is highly respected by his or her peers.

Surgeon's Credentials

Good credentials are a sign of a smart, hardworking, motivated surgeon. You should evaluate the potential surgeon's credentials before you visit his or her office. It is easy to find out these credentials on the Web. You can also call the doctor's office and ask for the doctor's resume or curriculum vitae (the traditional name for a doctor's resume). Alternatively, you can call the office and ask to speak to the refractive surgery coordinator. This person can answer questions about credentials on the phone.

Medical School

To perform eye surgery, a doctor has to have gone to medical school. Avoid U.S.-born surgeons who have attended medical school outside the United States. That means they likely weren't strong enough applicants to get admitted to an American medical school. On the other hand, there are some foreign-born doctors who went to medical school abroad and then moved to the United States. These can be excellent doctors because it is very hard for non-U.S.-born surgeons to get licensed in the United States if they trained abroad.

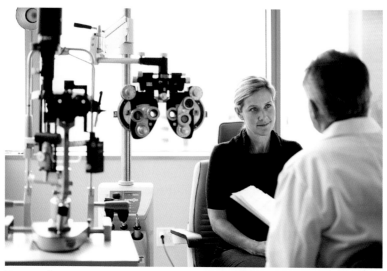

Your eyes deserve the most capable eye surgeon you can find. As you interview a prospective surgeon, it's important to find out how experienced the surgeon is in performing the type of procedure you wish to have.

Residency

Eye surgery is done by an ophthalmologist. An ophthalmologist is a medical doctor who has completed three years of specialized training in eye diseases and surgery. This training is called a residency. Look for a doctor who has gone to one of the top twenty residency programs. Generally, the top twenty programs attract the best medical students, and they also train them better than the other programs. You can find a ranking of eye hospitals at http://health.usnews.com/best-hospitals/rankings/ophthalmology. Although this is not an exact ranking of training programs, it is a useful guide.

Fellowship

Generally, the best doctors go on to do one or two more years of optional specialized training, called *fellowship training*. This specialized training can be done in different fields. Look for an ophthalmologist who has done fellowship training in either corneal surgery, refractive surgery, or cataract surgery. Fellowship-trained surgeons are generally more skilled and more experienced.

Membership in Professional Organizations

Being a member of professional organizations dedicated to refractive surgery can be a sign that the surgeon is committed to improving his or her knowledge in the field. Look for membership in the International Society of Refractive Surgery (ISRS) or the American Society of Cataract and Refractive Surgery (ASCRS). Membership, however, is not necessarily a great credential because pretty much anyone who is willing to pay the dues can join. The exception is the American-European Congress of Ophthalmic Surgery (AECOS), which can be joined by invitation only, and membership is limited to the top surgeons in North America and Europe.

Having a leadership role in one of these organizations is a strong credential. A leadership role could be an officer or a committee member in the organization. Generally, the leaders rose to their position because they have been capable surgeon innovators who are at the top of their field. Look for a surgeon who has been a program chairman or cochairman. These are the people who choose the subjects to be discussed at the national meetings. They have to know the field inside out to be selected for these positions.

Scientific Publications

There are a variety of professional journals and newspapers. Peer-reviewed journals have the highest standards. Every article is carefully reviewed for accuracy by two experts. Many articles are rejected. Getting an article published in one of these journals is difficult and is a strong sign of expertise.

Look for a surgeon who has published scientific articles in peer-reviewed journals. This is a sign of unusual commitment and deeper understanding of the field. Go to the National Library of Medicine website, called PubMed (www.ncbi.nlm.nih.gov/pubmed). Type in the prospective surgeon's last name, a hyphen and initials (Maloney-RK or Shamie-N for the authors) and hit search. Up will come a list of everything the surgeon has published in a peer-reviewed journal. More than twenty publications is a very strong credential.

There are also newspapers and magazines written for doctors that are less rigorous and more like easy reading. We call these throwaways because they aren't worth keeping on the bookshelf. Nearly any doctor who wants to can get an article published in one of these journals, so publication in these journals is not a strong credential. Popular throwaways include *Ocular Surgery News,* and *Advanced Ocular Care.* Go to the National Library of Medicine website to evaluate a surgeon's publications. If the journal is not listed there, it is a throwaway.

Participation in FDA Clinical Trials

The Food and Drug Administration (FDA) authorizes some ophthalmologists to participate as principal investigators in *clinical trials* sponsored by manufacturers. A clinical trial is a research study, conducted with patients, that is designed to evaluate the safety and effectiveness of a new drug or device. Typically, FDA-authorized ophthalmologists are chosen because of their demonstrated skill and their ability to get great results with refractive surgery. These surgeons are subject to detailed analysis and reporting and are willing to endure a high level of scrutiny. An ophthalmologist who has participated as a principal investigator in multiple FDA refractive surgery trials is likely to be an excellent surgeon for you.

Warning Signs

There are number of warning signs that a surgeon is not competent to perform your vision correction surgery. Take the time to make sure the surgeon you select does not fall into the following categories.

Lack of Board Certification

At the conclusion of their training, all newly minted eye doctors take a rigorous oral and written test of their knowledge. Those who pass this test are called *board certified.* Doctors who fail can take it again. Eventually, about 90 percent of eye doctors pass the test. That means that if a surgeon is not board certified, he or she was in the bottom 10 percent of their knowledge of the field. If you find an eye surgeon is non-board-certified, run the other way! To verify whether a specific eye doctor is board certified, you can go to the American Board of Medical Specialties (ABMS) website at www.abms.org. You can also check out the American Board of Ophthalmology website, http://abop.org/verify-a-physician, for the names of board-certified eye surgeons.

Excessive Number of Malpractice Suits

Even the best surgeons occasionally get sued for malpractice. We live in a culture where lawsuits are frequent. You want a surgeon with lots of experience, and lawsuits are, unfortunately, a part of any busy surgeon's experience. The typical vision correction surgeon is sued roughly once for every 3,000 surgeries performed. Statistics indicate that about 80 percent of these suits are either frivolous or without merit. Look for a surgeon with fewer than one lawsuit per 5,000 surgeries. If the doctor has been sued more frequently than this, or has multiple simultaneous lawsuits, you should ask for an explanation. If you are embarrassed to ask about malpractice suits against the doctor, there are alternative ways to obtain this information.

The Federation of State Medical Boards collects and disseminates information about doctors' malpractice histories. It takes five to seven days to get an answer to a request. Contact the organization at its website, www. fsmb.org. Many state medical boards offer lists of judgments against a doctor or settlements by the doctor. Check your state medical board's website.

Sanctions by the State Medical Board

All doctors must be licensed by the state medical board in any state in which they practice. Medical boards will discipline doctors for significant misbehavior, including gross or repeated acts of negligence. Contact your state medical board for information on the doctor you are considering. Many state medical boards now publish disciplinary actions against surgeons on-line. Medical boards are often criticized for being too lenient in disciplining physicians. A physician who has been disciplined usually has to have done something pretty bad.

Surgeon's Practice Style and Statistics

Once you have the names of qualified refractive surgeons with good reputations and credentials, the next step is to find out more about their practice style and how you relate to the surgeon. There are aspects of the surgeon's practice that you will learn when you visit his or her office. You should keep your eyes and ears open and ask direct questions to find out this information. You will also want to find out about costs.

How Are Your Questions Handled?

When you find a doctor with a promising reputation and solid credentials, call the office and ask to speak with the surgery coordinator or a staff member who can answer your questions. Don't be shy about asking penetrating questions. Vision correction surgeons understand that patients have many questions about them and about the procedure, and they should be prepared to answer the questions for you.

"Feel" of the Practice

Visit the office. It should feel right to you. If it is too quiet, the doctor may not be busy enough to have the experience you want in a surgeon. If it feels like a bus station, with long waits and people overflowing out the doors, they may be too busy to provide a high level of attention to examining you and planning your surgery.

Connection with the Surgeon

Avoid the "shopping mall" approach to surgery, where patients are shuffled through to the surgical suite without first having met with the surgeon. Most doctors have knowledgeable and compassionate staff to help perform tests and answer questions. However, it is also important to meet the surgeon and receive his or her personal evaluation before you decide to have the surgery.

Do you feel a connection with the surgeon? Do you trust the person? Is he patient or rushing to get to the next patient? Does she answer your questions in a way that you understand? I believe your connection to the surgeon is important and something that you should pay close attention to.

Some patients choose to see their regular eye doctor, an optometrist or ophthalmologist, for their preoperative and postoperative care. If you plan to do this, be sure your surgeon is comfortable working with your regular eye doctor. Although the majority of people have an uncomplicated postoperative course, you want to make sure your care provider will be able to recognize complications if they arise and can either treat you or refer you for treatment before more serious, long-term repercussions occur.

Focus of Practice

A Jack-of-all-trades is a master of none. Look for a surgeon whose practice specialty is refractive surgery or refractive and cataract surgery. If your surgeon is a member of American Academy of Ophthalmology, that organization's website, www.aao.org, lets you search for member eye doctors by city, state, and specialty (refractive surgery). The site lists doctors' practice focus, current professional activity, educational history and degrees, residency, fellowships, teaching positions, board certification, contact information, and often a website address.

Number of Vision Correction Procedures Performed

You want a surgeon who has performed your procedure over and over. Studies clearly show that more experienced surgeons have lower complication rates. If you are a candidate for LASIK or PRK, look for a surgeon who has done a minimum of 3,000 LASIK procedures. If the ICL is the right procedure for you, look for a surgeon who has done at least 300. If refractive lens exchange is your procedure, you want a surgeon who is a busy cataract surgeon, doing at least 300 cataracts a year and who is also an experienced LASIK surgeon because LASIK enhancement may be needed after RLE.

Tracking Statistics

If the surgeon has readily available statistics of the practice's results, he or she is most likely *benchmarking*, or tracking, outcomes of vision correction surgery.

Benchmarking is very important because it indicates the surgeon is concerned about achieving the best possible results over time. There is no mandatory central reporting database for tracking outcomes, unless a surgeon is participating in a sanctioned clinical trial. Therefore, a surgeon's doing benchmarking voluntarily indicates high personal standards of professionalism and performance.

Fortunately, outcomes can be predicted by using scientific data. Each surgeon achieves somewhat different results with the same procedure. The best surgeons track their own results and adjust the laser to optimize each patient's outcome based on the surgeon's personal results. This adjustment factor for the laser is called a *nomogram*. A nomogram takes into consideration the surgeon's own technique and the type of laser he or she uses. A well-developed nomogram allows the surgeon to more accurately program the laser for each patient, increasing the likelihood of perfect vision.

It takes about 3,000 surgeries for a surgeon who tracks outcomes to develop a nomogram. The reality is that most surgeons have not compiled personal statistics, for one of three reasons: first, they haven't done enough procedures; second, they aren't willing to do the labor-intensive work of entering large numbers of cases into a database; or third, they don't have the statistical knowledge necessary to analyze their results. This is unfortunate because it reduces patients' chances of achieving a perfect 20/20 result. Ask to see the surgeon's nomogram.

Surgeon's Success and Complication Rates

The surgeon should be able to give you the percentage of patients whose procedures result in 20/20 vision or better. It's normal for more than 80 percent of LASIK patients to achieve this level of vision. In fact, with wavefront-guided treatment, which uses newer diagnostic technology, most patients in a top practice today have a 95 percent chance of achieving 20/20 vision. With data based on 1,000 or more procedures, your surgeon should be able to tell your chances of achieving a good result with the chosen procedure and whether you will need an enhancement procedure. Ask what percentage of patients report significant complications. Less than 1 percent is acceptable. Keep in mind that most complications, if they do occur, can be managed by an experienced surgeon.

Percentage of Patients the Surgeon Turns Away

A conscientious surgeon will turn away about 10 to 15 percent of the patients he or she evaluates if the surgeon believes they are not good candidates for surgery. Be wary of a doctor who rarely advises a patient against the procedure. Many factors can make a patient a poor candidate for vision correction surgery. No doctor with high ethical standards will perform laser surgery on your eyes if you are not a good candidate.

Employee Turnover

Much of the success of surgery depends on outstanding support staff. Was the support staff happy and helpful? Had they worked there for a long time or is there a lot of turnover?

During your visit, ask the employees you meet how long they have worked there and whether they like their job.

Type of Laser Used

Make sure your doctor uses a newest-generation excimer laser that is capable of performing wavefront-guided treatment. Laser technology has improved dramatically over the past decade. State-of-the-art lasers now have *eye tracking,* which further improves the safety of the procedure. If your eye moves accidentally during the treatment, the laser automatically tracks, or follows, it. Make sure your surgeon uses an eye-tracking laser. State-of-the-art lasers enable surgeons to treat larger areas, minimizing the risk of night-vision disturbances.

The FDA website, www.fda.gov, has links to laser manufacturers' websites, where some maintain lists of doctors certified to use their machines. If your doctor is not listed, you may wish to contact the laser manufacturer directly. Verify that the doctor has been certified by the laser company to operate a particular machine, which means he or she took a required training course.

Cost of Surgery

Cost should not be the main factor in choosing a surgeon. First and foremost, seek out a surgeon who has a good reputation in the medical community and plenty of experience. If you are swayed by low cost, this may signal trouble for you down the road. Find the best-qualified surgeon you can. He or she should have high medical standards for patient care and should also offer comprehensive postoperative care. The surgeon should be willing to perform enhancement procedures if they are needed, as well as be available for any problems that might arise after surgery. Also, the surgeon's staff should be well trained and compassionate.

The cost of surgery varies from surgeon to surgeon. Generally, high-quality, all-laser wavefront-guided vision correction surgery runs between $2,500 and $3,600 per eye. Lens-based surgeries are more expensive. Be sure to ask whether the quoted per-eye cost includes preoperative and postoperative care, as well as enhancement procedures. Many practices can help you arrange low-interest or no interest financing, which makes high-quality surgery affordable for almost everyone.

Working with Your Regular Eye Doctor

Many eye doctors today offer vision correction surgery as an option for their patients who don't want to wear glasses or contact lenses. Your regular eye doctor should review the risks and complications of vision correction surgery with you and provide written material to further your education. He or she will often do the comprehensive eye examination to ensure your eyes are healthy, and then refer you to a capable surgeon.

You may have a choice of having your postoperative care performed by the surgeon (or another doctor on his staff) or your regular eye doctor.

Often, your regular eye doctor will provide routine postoperative care for you as well. This carefully coordinated sharing of care between the surgeon and your primary eye doctor is called *comanagement*. It offers you the advantage of a second expert who knows you well to oversee the process and ensure that you are satisfied with the results.

If you are traveling far to be treated by an expert surgeon, you will naturally want to have your eye doctor close to home take care of you. If the surgeon is located nearby, you may still wish to have your regular eye doctor provide your routine postoperative care.

After surgery, your regular eye doctor will check your vision and examine your eyes to ensure proper healing, and he or she can provide temporary eyeglasses or contact lenses if needed during the healing process. After you have healed, can also help you make the decision about whether or not enhancement is appropriate if your vision is not perfect. Your regular eye doctor will stay in close contact with the surgeon in case any difficulties arise during your postoperative course.

Making the Decision

Sometimes, no matter how much information you have gathered, the decision to choose one experienced surgeon over another comes down to your personal feelings. Personal chemistry is important. Choose someone with whom you feel comfortable—someone who is easy to talk to, friendly, and professional. Naturally, you also want a surgeon who listens to your questions, answers them completely, and asks you questions as well.

A good doctor-patient relationship is important. Likewise, the surgeon's support staff should be highly trained, competent, and caring. These are the people who will help support you through the procedure.

Once you feel comfortable with your decision, after you've carefully researched surgeons in your area, you're ready to undertake one of the most transformative experiences of your lifetime—the elimination of your dependency on glasses or contacts.

In Closing

Today, LASIK vision correction is the most popular refractive surgery performed. Its reputation is well deserved, as people discover that LASIK delivers great vision safely when it is performed by experienced, skilled surgeons. Perhaps more telling than the general public's enthusiasm for LASIK, however, is the widespread acceptance the procedure has gained among professionals in the fields of ophthalmology and optometry. In fact, more eye doctors have had LASIK on their own eyes than any other group of people.

What does the future hold for people who could benefit from laser vision correction? LASIK is a mature procedure. The wavefront-guided, all-laser technology is excellent. Improvements are happening only very slowly now. For the foreseeable future, LASIK will continue to be the procedure of choice for most people with low and moderate refractive errors. The ICL is recommended for high levels of nearsightedness, and the refractive lens exchange is recommended for higher levels of hyperopia.

The great unsolved problem is presbyopia. Currently, we treat it with monovision or multifocal implants. These approaches all work pretty well, but none are perfect. New lenses are in the pipeline for refractive lens exchange that, we hope, could allow a much greater range of clear vision, from miles away to the tip of your nose. We don't yet know how we'll solve the issue of presbyopia, but it is an area of active investigation. We predict that by 2030 we'll eliminate presbyopia as easily as we eliminate nearsightedness, farsightedness, and astigmatism today.

If you've read this book, you now know a lot about vision correction surgery. Thank you for joining us on a journey through this field. It is our life's passion, and we're honored that you let us share it with you. Vision correction surgery has been a life-changing experience for many, including our family, our patients, and us as surgeons. The decision to have surgery is an important one that ultimately only you can make. We hope to have given you information that will help you make a sound decision that will enrich your life and allow you to enjoy the newfound freedom you experience from improved vision.

Resources

American Academy of Ophthalmology (AAO)
P.O. Box 7424
San Francisco, CA 94120-7424
Phone: (415) 561-8500
www.aao.org

American Board of Medical Specialties (ABMS)
1007 Church Street, Suite 404
Evanston, IL 60201-5913
Phone verification on surgeons: (866) ASK-ABMS
Phone: (847) 491-9091
www.abms.org

American Optometric Association (AOA)
243 North Lindbergh Boulevard
St. Louis, MO 63141
Phone: (314) 991-4100
Toll-free: (800) 365-2219
www.aoa.org
Washington-area office
1505 Prince Street, Suite 300
Alexandria, VA 22314
Toll-free: (800) 365-2219
www.aoa.org

American Society of Cataract and Refractive Surgery (ASCRS)
4000 Legato Road, Suite 850
Fairfax, VA 22033
Phone: (703) 591-2220
www.ascrs.org

American Society of Cataract and Refractive Surgery (ASCRS) Eye Surgery Education Council
4000 Legato Road, Suite 700
Fairfax, VA 22033
Phone: (703) 591-2220
www.ascrs.org
www.eyesurgeryeducation.com

Federation of State Medical Boards (FSMB)
Federation Place
400 Fuller Wiser Road, Suite 300
Euless, TX 76039-3855
Phone: (817) 868-4000
www.fsmb.org

Food and Drug Administration (FDA)
5600 Fishers Lane (HFE-88)
Rockville, MD 20852
Phone: (888) INFO-FDA, (888) 463-6332
www.fda.gov

International Society of Refractive Surgery of the American Academy of Ophthalmology (ISRS/AAO)
P.O. Box 7424
San Francisco, CA 94120-7424
Phone: (415) 561-8500
www.isrs.org

National Eye Institute (NEI)
31 Center Drive
MSC 2510
Bethesda, MD 20892-3655
Phone: (301) 496-5248
www.nei.nih.gov

National Library of Medicine (NLM)
8600 Rockville Pike
Bethesda, MD 20894
Toll-free: (888) FIND-NLM, (888) 346-3656; (301) 594-5983
www.ncbi.nlm.nih.gov/pubmed

Glossary

20/20 vision: Normal visual acuity. The numbers indicate that the tested eye, twenty feet away from the eye chart, sees as well as a person with normal vision at the same distance.

A

ablation: Removal or vaporization of tissue with a laser.

accommodation: The eye's ability to change lens shape (by action of the ciliary muscle and zonules) in order to focus clearly on objects at various distances. As the lens becomes more rigid with age—a condition called *presbyopia*—it is less able to accommodate.

anterior chamber: Area between the cornea and the iris filled with aqueous humor.

aqueous humor: Clear, watery fluid that fills the anterior chamber of the eye; maintains intraocular pressure and nourishes the cornea, iris, and lens.

artificial tears: Sterile eyedrops used to lubricate the eyes the same way natural tears do.

astigmatism: Visual distortion caused by a cornea whose surface is elongated—like the side of a football—rather than curved like an arc on a sphere. Light rays enter the eye unequally and may produce two focal points on the retina.

autorefractor: A device, used to test refractive error, that emits a pinpoint beam of light, which reflects off the retina and measures the eye's response.

axis measurement: A measurement of the direction of astigmatism. The astigmatic cornea is oval in shape, and axis is the angle of the long direction of the oval above a horizontal line.

B

benchmarking: The process of tracking statistical outcomes for the purpose of predicting future outcomes. With LASIK, statistics from 1,000 or more procedures can provide a good basis for benchmarking.

best corrected vision/ best corrected visual acuity (BCVA): The best possible vision achieved with corrective eyeglass lenses.

biomicroscope: Also called a *slit lamp,* this is a microscope that projects a flattened beam of light into the eye for close examination of its internal structures.

board certified: A credential awarded to physicians who have undergone additional training and proved proficiency in an area by passing a rigorous examination. Ninety percent of ophthalmologists are board certified, so this credential is of limited value in distinguishing one ophthalmologist from another. If a surgeon is not board certified in ophthalmology, beware!

C

capsular bag: A thin membrane that forms the outermost layer of the crystalline lens, outside of the cortex and the nucleus.

capsule: *See* capsular bag.

cataract: Clouded area (opacity) of the eye's natural lens; caused by trauma, disease, or aging, or may be congenital.

central vision: In the visual field, the area of sharpest vision, used for reading and distinguishing detail and color. *See also* peripheral vision.

comanagement: An arrangement in which the surgeon does the surgery and the primary eye doctor does all or part of the preoperative or postoperative care. Ideally, comanagement offers the advantage of a second expert to oversee care and ensure the patient's satisfaction with the results.

cone: One of more than 7 million retinal photoreceptor cells (in each eye) concentrated in the center of the retina, responsible for sharp vision and ability to see colors.

conjunctiva: Clear mucous membrane that covers the white of the eye (sclera) and lines the inner surface of the eyelids.

cornea: The outer, dome-shaped, transparent part of the eye that bulges out at the front of the eyeball and covers the iris and pupil. Its curvature causes light to bend. The cornea provides most of the eye's focusing power. It is the only part of the eye on which LASIK is performed.

corneal edema: Abnormal fluid buildup and consequent swelling of the cornea.

corneal pachymetry: Measurement of corneal thickness using ultrasound.

corneal topographer: An instrument that creates a three-dimensional map of the cornea, using computerized analysis.

corneal topography: Rendering of a precise three-dimensional map of the cornea using sophisticated camera and computer technology.

cortex: Soft, clear tissue that forms the middle layer of the crystalline lens between the capsule and the nucleus.

crystalline lens: The eye's natural lens; a flexible, transparent tissue, located behind the iris, that helps focus rays of light onto the retina. As the lens becomes less flexible with age, its ability to adapt its focus for reading gradually decreases, requiring the use of reading glasses. *See* presbyopia.

cylinder: One of three measures in an eyeglass prescription. It indicates whether astigmatism is present, and to what degree.

D

diabetes mellitus: A group of diseases that develop when the body is unable to use blood sugar for energy, causing excessive amounts of sugar in the bloodstream (hyperglycemia).

diopter: A measurement of how strong a lens is. Thicker lenses have a higher number of diopters. In eye care, it is used to measure your refractive error, or what eyeglass lens is needed to correct your vision. Hyperopia is measured in terms of positive diopters. Myopia is measured in terms of negative diopters.

disease neutral: Something that neither prevents diseases nor affects the treatment of diseases. LASIK is considered disease neutral.

dry eye: A condition characterized by corneal dryness due to inadequate tear production.

E

emmetropes: People who have no refractive error; that is, no nearsightedness, farsightedness, or astigmatism. Perfect refractive ability is referred to as *emmetropia.*

endophthalmitis: A serious infection, usually bacterial, of the interior of the eye.

endothelium: The innermost layer of the cornea, a single cell thick, that helps regulate the cornea's hydration

enhancement procedure: A secondary treatment with the excimer laser to fine-tune visual acuity after the initial LASIK procedure. Enhancements take place after vision has stabilized, usually three to six months after LASIK. Enhancements usually do not require making a new corneal flap.

epi-LASIK: A variant of PRK in which the epithelium (the clear skin that covers the eye) is peeled off by an automated machine called an *epikeratome.* The results are the same as with PRK.

epithelial ingrowth: A potential complication of LASIK produced when corneal surface cells, or epithelium, grow underneath the corneal flap during the first month after surgery. The condition is often easily diagnosed and treated.

epithelium: The thin, protective outermost surface of the cornea. It is made up of the same kind of cells that cover most of the body. The epithelium grows rapidly and continually regenerates.

excimer laser: The type of laser used in refractive surgery to remove corneal tissue. It emits highly precise pulses of ultraviolet light to break up tissue one molecular layer at a time, vaporizing it without generating heat that could damage surrounding tissue.

extended-range lens implant: A type of multifocal implant that gives good distance and intermediate vision. It generally gives sharper distance vision than other multifocal implants, but reading vision that is not as sharp.

eyelid: Thin, retractable tissue covering the front of the eye. The eyelid serves to protect the eye from dust and other foreign objects and from exceedingly bright light. It also distributes moisture (tears) over the cornea.

eyelid speculum: A device placed between the upper and lower eyelids to keep the patient from blinking during surgery. It is painless, because the eye is anesthetized.

F

farsightedness: *See* hyperopia.

field of vision: *See* visual field.

floaters: Particles in the vitreous humor that drift across the visual field.

Food and Drug Administration (FDA): The federal agency that regulates the manufacturers and distributors of drugs and devices. There is a popular misconception that the FDA regulates the practice of medicine. It does not; regulation of the practice of medicine is left up to the states. A related misconception is that the FDA approves medical and surgical procedures. It does not; the majority of medical and surgical procedures done in the United States are not FDA approved but rather are off-label, or unapproved.

fovea, fovea centralis: Central concave area of the macula that is packed with photoreceptors called cones, which produce the sharpest vision.

fundus: Interior surface of the back of the eyeball, visible with an ophthalmoscope. The eye's fundus includes the retina (with macula and fovea) and the juncture of the optic nerve with the eye.

G

glaucoma: Group of diseases usually associated with increased intraocular pressure; if untreated, can lead to blindness.

H

halo: Perceived rings around light sources viewed at night; often accompanied by starburst. A common symptom of cataracts.

haptics: The side struts, or extensions, on an intraocular lens that help to hold it in place after implantation.

haze: Scarring of the corneal stroma, or corneal bed. Significant haze occurs rarely after PRK, and does not occur after LASIK.

herpes simplex: A recurrent viral infection of the eye characterized by a painful sore on the eyelid or surface of the eye. It causes inflammation of the cornea and can lead to blindness. This is not a sexually transmitted infection. Patients with herpes simplex of the eye may not be candidates for LASIK.

higher-order aberration: Irregularity of vision that cannot be corrected by glasses or contact lenses.

hyperopia: Also known as *farsightedness,* hyperopia occurs when the eyeball is too short from front to back or when the eye's focusing mechanism is too weak, causing light rays to be focused behind, rather than on, the retina. People with hyperopia see objects at a distance more clearly than close up but usually have difficulty with both distance and near vision.

I

informed consent: A legal form a patient is asked to sign that thoroughly discusses the risks, benefits, alternative options, and possible complications of a surgical procedure.

intraocular lens (IOL): A synthetic lens implanted during refractive lens exchange to replace the natural lens.

intraocular pressure (IOP): The pressure exerted by the fluid within the eye that gives it its firmness and round shape.

IOL: *See* intraocular lens.

IOP: *See* intraocular pressure.

iris: The colored ring of tissue in the eye that is behind the cornea and in front of the lens. The muscles of the iris can adjust the size of the eye's opening, or pupil, to allow for larger or smaller amounts of light to enter the eye.

K

keratectomy: Surgical removal of any part of the cornea. In the context of LASIK, keratectomy is the flap-making part of the procedure.

keratomileusis: Any process of carving, or reshaping, the cornea.

L

lamellar: An adjective meaning *layered*. Lamellar corneal surgery corrects focusing errors by removing or reshaping some of the corneal layers.

Glossary

LASEK: Another name for PRK.

laser: Acronym for light amplification by stimulated emission of radiation, a high-energy light source used medically to cut, burn, or dissolve tissues.

LASIK: An acronym for laser *in-situ* keratomileusis. In LASIK, either a laser or mechanical vibrating blade creates a very thin, hinged flap on the surface of the cornea. After the flap is gently lifted back, the surgeon reshapes the corneal stroma, using an excimer laser. The corneal flap is then replaced, and it quickly adheres. LASIK is a safe and pain-free form of refractive eye surgery that has proven to be highly successful and popular.

legal blindness: Visual acuity of 20/200 or worse with glasses.

lens: *See* crystalline lens.

limbal-relaxing incisions: A technique for correcting astigmatism. Small incisions are made in the limbus—the thin connection between the cornea and the white of the eye (the sclera)—that cause the cornea to become more rounded.

M

macula: Small central area of the retina filled with light-sensitive photoreceptors called *rods* and *cones.*

macular degeneration: A progressive eye disease caused by deterioration of the central portion of the retina, called the *macula.*

microkeratome: The instrument that was traditionally used by a surgeon to create the corneal flap in the uppermost layer of the cornea during the LASIK procedure. In modern LASIK, the flap is made with a laser.

monofocal intraocular lens: A lens implant that has a single, fixed focal point. The focus can be set for distance, intermediate, or near vision. Eyeglasses or monovision are needed for good vision at other distances.

monovision: A process by which a surgeon corrects one eye for seeing at a distance and the other eye for seeing objects close up.

multifocal intraocular lens: A lens implant that provides good near and distance vision without glasses.

myopia: Nearsightedness, occurring when the eye is too long and images come into focus before they reach the retina. A nearsighted person, or myope, may have good near vision but have difficulty seeing objects at a distance.

N

nearsightedness: *See* myopia.

nomogram: The surgeon's formula that is entered into the laser's computer calculation to further refine the manufacturer's recommended settings.

O

ophthalmologist: A medical doctor who specializes in the diagnosis and medical or surgical treatment of eye disorders and disease.

ophthalmology: The field of medicine dealing with diseases and surgery of the eye.

ophthalmoscope: An illuminated instrument used to examine structures in the back of the eye.

optic nerve: A bundle of nerve fibers, about the diameter of a pencil, that connect to the nerve fiber layer of the retina and terminate in the brain. The optic nerve carries the visual messages from the photoreceptors of the retina to the brain, where images are created and processed.

optician: One who is trained to fit and dispense eyeglasses and, in some states, contact lenses, according to a prescription from an optometrist or ophthalmologist.

optometrist: An eye care professional specializing in the examination, diagnosis, treatment, management, and prevention of diseases and disorders of the eye. Optometrists do not perform surgery, but otherwise perform most functions that ophthalmologists do. Optometrists are often general eye care providers and can provide preoperative and postoperative care for LASIK patients and other refractive surgery patients.

orbit: The bony socket that surrounds the eyeball.

overcorrection: The amount of correction resulting from the LASIK or other procedure that is more than intended. Normally this is treated with an enhancement procedure.

P

pachymetry: Measurement of corneal thickness.

Glossary

peripheral vision: Side vision; in the visual field, perception of objects outside the direct line of vision. *See also* central vision.

phoropter: An eye-examination device consisting of a complete range of corrective lenses that can be adjusted to hundreds of combinations, which the patient is asked to evaluate. By continually changing the lenses, the doctor can arrive at a combination of lens strengths that becomes the basis of a prescription for corrective lenses.

photoablation: The process of removing, or vaporizing, tissue by means of laser energy.

photoreceptor cells: Light-sensitive cells—rods and cones—on the retina that allow the eye to see in dim light, distinguish colors, and perceive contrast.

photorefractive keratectomy (PRK): A type of laser vision correction that reshapes the cornea by ablating, or vaporizing, the corneal tissue one microscopic layer at a time, using an excimer laser. Unlike LASIK, in which a hinged corneal flap is first made and lifted back to expose the corneal bed, with PRK the sculpting is done on the outer layer of the cornea.

posterior capsule: The rear part of the lens capsule, which is left in place during refractive lens exchange to help support the implanted lens.

posterior capsule opacification: An opacity that can develop on the posterior capsule after lens replacement. It is treated in the office with a YAG laser.

posterior chamber: The fluid-filled area between the iris and the lens.

presbyopia: Often confused with farsightedness, presbyopia (literally, "old eyes") is the age-dependent need for reading glasses or bifocals, caused by the decreasing ability of the eye's lens and surrounding muscles to fine-tune focus.

prescription: A series of numbers that instruct someone how to provide a patient with the proper eyeglass or contact lens (*See also* refractive error).

punctal plugs: Used in the treatment of dry eye, these tiny silicone plugs are inserted into the tear-drainage openings of the eyelid to delay the drainage of natural tears so the eyes will stay moist.

pupil: Black circular opening in the center of the iris. Through muscular action of the iris, the pupil constricts or dilates to regulate the amount of light that enters the eye.

R

radial keratotomy (RK): A form of refractive surgery in which the surgeon alters the shape of the cornea by making thin incisions around it in a spokelike pattern. The incisions cause the central portion of the cornea to flatten, treating myopia and astigmatism. RK is no longer performed.

refract: To bend, as when light passes through a curved shape such as a cornea or lens.

refraction: Bending of light as it passes from one material to another. Also, a test to determine the eye's refractive error.

refractive error: The eyeglass prescription needed to correct your vision. Refractive error has three parts: sphere (how nearsighted or farsighted you are), cylinder (how much astigmatism you have), and axis (the angle of your astigmatism).

refractive lens exchange (RLE): Like cataract surgery, a procedure to remove the crystalline lens and replace it with a synthetic lens. Refractive lens exchange, however, is performed before cataracts have developed significantly, generally because the patient cannot or does not wish to wear eyeglasses or contact lenses.

refractive surgery: Any type of surgery that changes the focusing power of the eye in order to correct a refractive error. LASIK is a type of refractive surgery that corrects the eye's focusing ability by reshaping the curvature of the cornea.

retina: The light-sensitive layer of cells on the inner back surface of the eye that processes light and functions much like film in a camera. The retina converts light into electrical impulses, which are transmitted along the optic nerve to the brain, which in turn interprets the impulses as images.

retinal detachment: Separation of the retina from the underlying pigment epithelium, requiring urgent surgery to correct

retinal pigment epithelium: The part of the retina consisting of dark tissue cells that absorb excess light and carry nutrients to, and waste products from, the retina

rod: One of more than 120 million retinal photoreceptor cells (in each eye) that are especially receptive to brightness and allow us to see in dim light.

S

sclera: The tough white part of the eye that makes up five-sixths of the outer layer of the eyeball. Along with the cornea, it protects the eyeball.

Snellen eye chart: Standard assessment instrument for visual acuity; chart consisting of rows of letters (largest at the top, smallest at the bottom) developed by Dutch ophthalmologist Hermann Snellen in 1862; usually read at a distance of twenty feet.

socket: *See* orbit.

sphere: One of three measurements taken during an eye examination to arrive at one's eyeglass prescription. The sphere measures where the eye focuses light—on the retina (normal vision), in front of the retina (myopia), or behind the retina (hyperopia).

starburst: A visual aberration in which the patient sees rays radiating from lights viewed at night. Starbursts are seen by everyone, even those who haven't had refractive surgery. Refractive surgery can increase the amount of starburst the patient perceives.

striae: Wrinkles or folds in the corneal flap after LASIK. Small striae, called microstriae, usually do not affect vision. Larger striae, or macrostriae, can be smoothed out easily.

stroma: The strong, fibrous layer that makes up 90 percent of the cornea's thickness and provides the cornea with its structure and shape. Also called the *stromal bed,* this is the part of the cornea sculpted with the laser in LASIK and PRK surgery.

T

tear: Thin film of fluid that lubricates the front of the eye. Blinking spreads tear film evenly across the surface.

tonometer: A device that measures intraocular pressure, or the pressure inside the eye.

toric lens implant: A lens implant specially designed to correct astigmatism.

U

ultraviolet (UV) light: Electromagnetic radiation, shorter in wavelength than visible radiation but longer than X-rays.

undercorrection: The amount of correction resulting from the LASIK procedure that is less than intended. Most undercorrections can be treated with an enhancement procedure.

V

visual acuity: The sharpness or clarity of vision that enables one to distinguish fine details and shapes.

visual field: Extent of the area visible to an eye looking straight ahead; includes central and peripheral vision.

vitrectomy: Surgical removal of the vitreous, which is replaced with clear fluid.

vitreous, vitreous humor: Clear gel-like substance that fills the rear two-thirds of the eyeball between the lens and the retina.

W

wavefront analyzer: A device that uses laser light rays to measure irregularities in the focusing power of the eye. This data can be fed into the laser during LASIK and PRK procedures to correct vision to better than 20/20.

Y

YAG laser: Yttrium aluminum garnet laser, which produces a short-pulse, high-energy light beam to cut or perforate tissue. It is used to treat posterior capsule opacification.

Z

zonule: The fibers that connect the ciliary muscle to the crystalline lens. Contraction and relaxation of the ciliary muscle change the tension of the fibers, which in turn changes the focusing power of the eye. The fibers also help to hold the lens in place.

Index

Numbers

20/15 vision, 42, 44
20/20 vision, 12, 18, 34, 42, 51, 53, 119
20/40 vision, 34, 52, 53

A

ablation of tissue, 17
accommodating IOL, 16
Accutane, 30
aching pain in eyeball, 91
acne medications, 30
acuity test, 34
Advanced Ocular Care, 115
allergies, 30
all-laser LASIK, 16, 18, 42, 46, 47, 58, 121
  advantages, 42
  costs, 120
all-laser wavefront-guided technology, 64
American Academy of Ophthalmology, 118
American Board of Medical Specialties (ABMS), 115
American Board of Ophthalmology, 115
American Society of Cataract and Refractive Surgery (ASCRS), 114
American-European Congress of Ophthalmic Surgery (AECOS), 114
America's Top Doctors, 112
anesthesia, 46, 70
anesthesiologist, 86, 103, 104
anesthetic eyedrops, 47, 71, 79
anterior segment, 35
  examination, 35
antibiotic eyedrops, 60, 74, 87, 92
antibiotic injections, 108
anti-inflammatory eyedrops, 50, 87, 108
anxiety, 46
arthritis, 30
artificial tears, 50
asthma, 30
astigmatism, 121
autoimmune diseases, 29, 30
axis measurements, 13, 14

B

bacteria, 60, 88, 92, 104, 105
bandage contact lens, 59, 71, 72
  removal, 72
basement membrane, 40, 69
basement membrane dystrophy, 40
benchmarking, 118
Best Doctors in America, 112
bifocal glasses, 8, 11, 12, 14, 21
biocompatibility, 83, 84
biomicroscope, 35
birth defects, 29

blade LASIK, 16, 18
blade-fee LASIK, 42
blood pressure, 104
blood vessels, 35
blurry vision, 4, 5, 6, 56, 60, 65, 70, 76, 78, 79, 90, 108
board certification of surgeon, 118
breast milk, 29
breastfeeding, 29
burning eyes, 61

C

capsular bag, 104, 107
cataract surgery, 3, 99, 100, 113, 118
Cataract Surgery: A Patient's Guide to Cataract Treatment, 3
cataracts, 14, 21, 30, 40, 63, 80, 82, 85, 92, 99, 100, 102
advantages of RLE, 100, 101
central vision, 107
clarity of vision, 107
clinical trials, 115, 118
close range vision, 9, 10, 11, 24, 90
collagen, 83, 84
comanagement, 121
complication rates, 118
complications possible with ICL, 89–93
complications possible with LASIK, 55–60
complications possible with PRK, 75–78
comprehensive eye examination, 32, 33–36, 42, 56, 62, 63, 69, 81, 121
contact lens, 2, 5
contact lens prescriptions, 32
contact lenses, 7, 8, 15, 41, 42, 43, 56, 60, 62
prior to preoperative evaluation, 32

removal prior to eye surgery, 87, 103
cornea, 2, 17, 21, 23, 32, 35, 41, 66, 67, 83
abrasions, 40, 41
curvature, 4, 6, 15, 37, 38
diseases, 35
oval-shape, 97
reshaping, 18, 37, 39, 47, 48, 49, 65, 68, 71
scaring, 60, 63
thin, 63, 67, 73, 85
tissue removal from periphery, 67
weak, 40
cornea surgery, 16
cornea-based refractive surgery, 15–19
corneal abrasions, 40, 41, 57, 69
after LASIK, 40
from contact lenses, 41
from trauma, 41
corneal crosslinking, 60
corneal ectasia, 59, 60, 78
corneal epithelial defect, 57
see also corneal abrasions, 57
corneal flap, 37, 49, 50, 58, 61, 76
see also LASIK flap, 37
wrinkles, 58, 59
corneal haze, 76, 82
corneal inlays, 16, 23
corneal surgery, 113
current medications, 32, 86, 103
cylinder, 13
cylinder measurements, 13

D

depth of penetration, 78
diabetes complications, 30
diabetic retinopathy, 30
dietary supplements, 57
dilation of the pupil, 36, 87, 104
diopers, 39, 54, 55, 68, 85

Index

distance range vision, 7, 8, 9, 10, 11, 12, 21, 23, 24, 39
driving after procedure, 46
driving at night, 57
dry eyes, 29
  testing, 35, 56, 62
  treatment options, 57
dusty environments, 51, 74, 105
dysphotopsia, 107

E

enhancement procedure, 28, 51, 52, 54, 55, 56, 61, 62, 76, 90, 119
  after PRK, 75
  costs, 120
  recovery, 52
epi-LASIK, 66
  see PRK (photorefractive keratectomy)
epithelial ingrowth, 59, 76
epithelium, 17, 18, 40, 41, 59, 67, 69
  healing after surgery, 74
  recurrent erosions, 76
  removal, 66, 71
  slips, 76
excimer laser, 17, 18, 19, 37, 38, 39, 42, 44, 47, 48, 61, 65, 67, 120
extended range lens implant, 97, 98
  disadvantages, 98
extreme myopia, 77
eye diseases, 28, 63, 82, 113
eye examination,
  see comprehensive eye examination
eye health, 28
eye history, 32
eye hospital ratings, 113
eye measurements, 32
eye pressure, 30, 91
eye surgeon, 110–122

board certification, 118
  choosing, 110–122
  complication rates, 119
  credentials, 110, 112, 116
  curriculum vitae, 112
  degrees, 118
  educational history, 118
  employee turnover, 119
  excessive malpractice suits, 116
  experience, 110
  fellowship training, 113
  focus of practice, 118
  Internet research, 111
  lack of board certification, 115
  medical school, 112
  memberships in professional organizations, 114
  number of precedures performed, 118
  online reviews, 111
  participation in FDA clinical trials, 115
  patient referrals, 110, 111
  percentage of patients turned away, 119
  practice style, 110, 111, 116–120
  qualifications, 110
  ratings, 112
  reputation, 110, 116, 117
  residency, 113, 118
  resume, 112
  review websites, 112
  sanctions by state medical board, 116
  scientific publications, 114
  statistics, 118
  success rates, 119
  teaching positions, 118
  tracking statistics, 118
  warning signs, 115
eye surgery centers, 32, 64
eye tracking, 120
eyeglass prescriptions, 13, 53,

55, 68
eyeglasses, glasses, 3, 7, 15, 28, 32, 42, 43, 45, 73
eyelid speculum, 47, 49, 71
eyelids, 35, 91
  inflammation, 35

F

farsightedness, 3, 6, 16, 18, 19, 21, 25, 28, 39, 54, 66, 67, 68, 75, 77, 85, 90, 95, 98, 108, 121
FDA clinical trials, 115
FDA study, 58, 92
Federation of State Medical Boards, 116
femtosecond laser, 18, 42
flapless LASIK, 66
  see PRK (photorefractive keratectomy)
focus, 2, 3, 4, 6, 9, 25, 38
focusing problems, 3
follow-up appointments, 60, 88
Food and Drug Administration (FDA), 120
friends and family members, 33

G

glasses,
  see eyeglasses, glasses
  for night driving, 24
glaucoma, 35, 63, 82

H

halos, 28, 44, 45, 50, 54, 90, 91
haptics, 96
Hashimoto's thyroiditis, 29
hazy vision, 49, 54, 71, 100
hereditary conditions, 40
herpes keratitis, 40
  reactivation from LASIK, 40
high astigmatism, 14, 58
high myopia, 58
higher-order aberrations, 43, 44
highly hyperopic, 14
highly myopic, 14
hyperopia, 4, 6, 12, 19, 21, 28,

39, 43, 44, 54, 55, 68

I

ICL possible complications, 89–93
  cataracts, 92
  halos, 90
  overcorrection, 90
  presbyopia, 90
  starburst, 90
  undercorrection, 90
immune system, 29, 84
implantable contact lens (ICL), 5, 7, 16, 19, 20, 21, 22, 23, 39, 54, 58, 63, 68, 83–94, 95, 118
  advantages, 83, 84
  advantages over LASIK, 84
  advantages over PRK, 84
  astigmatism, 85
  driving day of surgery, 88
  enhancement procedure, 90
  FAQs, 93, 94
  implantation procedure, 86, 87
  monovision, 90
  next-day checkup, 87
  poor candidates for procedure, 85
  postoperative care, 88
  preoperative instructions, 86
  rare complications, 92
  recovery, 21, 85, 87, 88
  removal, 91
  results to expect, 89
  resuming activity after procedure, 88
  safety advantages, 89
  sizes, 92
incisional corneal surgeries, 22
infection, 35, 74, 88, 103, 105, 108
inflammation, 53
informed consent, 36
initial consultation, 32
intermediate vision, 11, 24

Index

International Society of Refractive Surgery (ISRS), 114
Internet research, 111
intraocular lens implant (IOL), 95, 96
implant choices, 96–99
types, 96, 97
intraocular pressure measurement, 35
iris, 2, 3, 35, 83

K

keratoconus, 18, 40, 59, 67, 78

L

lamellar refractive surgery, 63, 81, 82
LASEK, 66
see PRK (photorefractive keratectomy)
laser, 42, 108
see also excimer laser
type used, 120
laser surgery, 17
LASIK (laser in-situ keratomileusis), 5, 7, 16, 19, 22, 23, 25, 34, 37–65, 93, 111, 119
advances, 13
after ICL procedure, 90
astigmatism, 39
benefits, 54
candidates for, 15, 37, 39, 63
complications, 37, 51, 55–60
conditions for poor candidates, 39–41
contact lenses, 63
differences from PRK, 65
discomfort after procedure, 61
driving after procedure, 51, 62
driving restrictions, 46
dry eyes, 35, 41, 49, 56, 62
enhancement procedure, 62
FAQs, 61–64
follow-up appointments, 51

hazy vision after surgery, 49
hyperopic correction, 38
and myopic correction, 37, 38
next-day checkup, 49
poor candidates for procedure, 55
postoperative care, 50, 51
presbyopia, 39
procedure, 46–49
recovery, 18, 41, 49, 50, 61, 65
reshaping the cornea, 38
results to expect, 51–55
resuming activity after procedure, 51
returning to work, 62
risk factors, 54
seeing better than 20/20, 42
side effects, 35, 44
statistics, 52
surgery on both eyes, 64
tracking statistics, 52
undergoing procedure, 46
visual stability, 50
LASIK enhancement, 106
LASIK flap, 16, 17, 37, 38, 40, 41, 42, 48, 59, 78
complications, 76
see also corneal flap
LASIK possible complications
corneal abrasions, 57
corneal ectasia, 59
corneal flap issues, 58
dry eyes, 56
epithelial ingrowth, 59
halos, 57, 58
infection, 60
overcorrection, 56
quality of vision issues, 58
starburst, 57, 58
undercorrection, 56
LASIK surgeon, 15, 61
see also eye surgeons
LASIK touch-up procedure, 89
legal blindness, 35

lens, 2, 3, 4, 6, 14, 35
  replacement, 5
  weakness, 6
lens-based refractive surgery, 15,
  19–23
light refraction, 4
light-adjustable lens (LAL)
  implant, 97, 98, 103, 106
limbal relaxing incisions, 22, 23
lubricating eyedrops, 49, 50, 53,
  57, 61
lupus, 29, 30

M
macula,
  fluid accumulation, 108
macular degeneration, 14, 35,
  63, 82
magnifying glasses, 105
makeup, 51, 70, 74, 86, 88, 92,
  103, 105
  using old, 60, 88
Manche, Dr. Edward, 44
medical conditions, 29
medical eye history, 32
microkeratome, 17, 18, 41, 58
  limitations, 41, 42
mild astigmatism, 14
mild farsightedness, 14
mild nearsightedness, 14
military services, 31, 93
mitomycin C, 82
moderate astigmatism, 14
moderate farsightedness, 14
moderate nearsightedness, 14
monofocal lens implant, 97
monofocal lenses, 25
monovision, 24, 25, 39, 50, 62,
  73, 81, 89, 90, 98, 106, 121
  testing, 24
multifocal lens implant, 16, 25,
  26, 97, 98, 99, 105, 106, 107,
  121
  disadvantages, 98

multifocal lens implants, 7, 25,
  26
myopia, 4, 5, 11, 19, 27, 28, 37,
  39, 43, 44, 55, 58, 63, 89
  causes, 4, 5
  see also nearsightedness

N
National Library of Medicine,
  114, 115
natural lens, 21, 22, 23, 87, 95,
  97, 107
Navy Medical Center,
  San Diego study, 44, 45
near vision, 9, 11, 23, 24, 25, 77
nearsightedness, 3, 5, 16, 18, 19,
  20, 37, 38, 39, 58, 66, 75, 76,
  77, 85, 87, 90, 92, 96, 98, 121
  see also myopia
nerve damage, 36
nerve fibers, 3
night driving, 24, 98, 106, 107
night vision, 57, 89, 91
night-vision disturbances, 28, 44,
  45, 57, 107
nomogram, 118, 119
non-laser cornea-based
  refractive surgery, 16
nonsteroidal anti-inflammatory
  (NSAID) eyedrops, 72, 74
normal vision, 1, 3, 4, 42
  see also 20/20 vision
normal visual acuity, 12
  see also 20/20 vision
numbing eyedrops, 46, 61, 65,
  70, 72, 74, 87, 109

O
occupational factors, 30, 31
Ocular Surgery News, 115
old makeup, 60
ophthalmologist, 14, 30, 34, 44,
  45, 68, 88, 113, 117
ophthalmology, 30, 121
ophthalmoscope, 36

Index

optic nerve, 2, 3
  examination, 35
optometrist, 111, 117
  referrals, 111
optometry, 121
oral corticosteroids, 30
oral pain relievers, 72
oral sedatives, 29, 46, 70
overcorrection, 56
over-the-counter medications, 30, 32

P

patient expectations, 31
peripheral iridotomy, 86, 88, 91
  driving after procedure, 86
  enlargement procedure, 91
  prior to ICL placement procedure, 86
  treatment to enlarge, 88
phoropter, 42
photorefractive keratectomy (PRK),
  see PRK (photorefractive keratectomy)
pneumonia, 86
posterior capsule, 108
  breakage, 108
posterior capsule opacification, 107, 108
postoperative care, 117, 120
postoperative discomfort, 61, 79
postoperative instructions, 60
prednisone, 30
pregnancy, 29
  vision changes during, 29
preoperative care, 117, 120
preoperative consultation, 33
preoperative evaluation, 32–36, 55
preoperative examinations, 28, 40, 59
presbyopia, 7–9, 11, 12, 14, 15, 23, 24, 25, 26, 89, 100, 121

causes, 9
and farsightedness, 12
and nearsightedness, 11
prescription medications, 30
previous eye surgeries, 28, 33, 63, 81
prior episodes of herpes keratitis, 40
PRK (photorefractive keratectomy), 5, 7, 18, 22, 39, 40, 63, 65–82
  20/20 vision, 74
  advantages over LASIK, 76
  astigmatism, 67
  basement membrane dystrophy, 69
  candidates for, 67–70, 81
  cataracts, 69
  compared to LASIK, 78
  complications, 75
  contact lenses after surgery, 81
  corneal ectasia, 78
  degree of refractive error, 68
differences from LASIK, 65
  discomfort after procedure, 79
  driving after procedure, 70, 80
  dry eyes, 35, 69, 77, 81
  enhancement procedure, 75, 76, 80, 81
  FAQs, 79
  halos, 78
  healing after surgery, 79
  hyperopic correction, 67
  keratoconus, 68, 69
  managing discomfort, 72
  myopic correction, 66, 67
  next-day checkup, 74
  overcorrection, 77
  phases of recovery, 72–74
  postoperative care, 74
  preoperative instructions, 70
  previous eye surgeries, 81
  prior episodes of herpes virus, 69

147

procedure, 66, 70, 71
quality of vision problems, 77
recovery, 18, 65, 72–74
recurrent erosions of epithelium, 76
results to expect, 74, 75
resuming activity after procedure, 74
returning to work, 80
risk factors, 75
side effects, 35
starburst, 78
statistics, 75
surgery on both eyes, 73, 82
thin cornea, 81
tracking statistics, 75
visual stability, 73
wavefront-guided PRK, 70, 82
PRK possible complications, 75–78
corneal haze, 76
undercorrection, 76
PRK touch-up procedure, 89
pupil, 2, 3, 91
unusually large, 28
size, 28, 29
night vision, 28

Q
quality of vision, 58, 77, 84, 89

R
radical keratotomy (RK)
see RK (radial keratotomy)
range of correction, 78
range of vision, 9, 10
close range vision, 10
distance range vision, 10
intermediate vision, 10
reading glasses, 7, 8, 11, 23, 28, 50, 62, 76, 89, 90, 105
reading vision, 7, 12, 15, 21, 39, 80
recovery of vision, 78
recovery room, 104

recurrent erosions, 76
refractive error, 3-7, 13, 15, 42, 43, 52, 56, 76
refractive lens exchange (RLE), 5, 7, 16, 21, 22, 23, 25, 39, 40, 55, 68, 69, 85, 95–109
advantages, 100, 101
benefits, 25
candidates for, 102
driving after procedure, 105
FAQs, 109
postoperative care, 105
potential complications, 106–109
preoperative instructions, 102
procedure, 102–104
recovery, 104, 105
results to expect, 105, 106
resuming activity after procedure, 105
side effects, 106
swimming, surfing, hot tubs, 105
refractive surgeons,
see eye surgeons
refractive surgery, 15, 113, 118
types of procedures, 16
refractive surgery coordinator, 112
regular eye doctor, 117, 121
relaxing incisions, 7
see also limbal relaxing incisions
residency programs, 113
retina, 2, 4, 5, 12, 37, 108
examination, 35
retinal camera, 36
retinal detachment, 63, 82, 108
retinal detachment surgery, 108
rheumatoid arthritis, 29
riboflavin eyedrops, 60
RK (radial keratotomy), 16, 22, 63, 81
RLE possible complications

Index

floaters, 108
halos, 107
posterior capsule opacification, 107, 108
residual farsightedness, 106
residual nearsightedness, 106
retinal detachment, 108
  shadows from edge of implant, 107
  starburst, 107
rubbing eyes, 50, 59, 74

S

sclera, 2, 5, 21, 47, 83, 87
sedation, 87, 109
sedatives, 49, 50, 62, 80, 104
seeing rings around lights, 26
severe dry eye, 29
single focus IOL, 16, 25
Snellen, Hermann, 34
Snellen eye chart, 4, 5, 6, 34, 35
sphere, 13
sphere measurements, 13, 54
stable eyeglass prescription, 28, 39
standard lens implant, 97
Stanford University, 44
starburst, 28, 30, 44, 45, 50, 54, 55, 57, 90, 91
steroid anti-inflammatory eyedrops, 74, 88
striae, 58, 59, 76
stroma, 17, 18, 37, 41, 66
subclinical keratoconus, 59
sunglasses, after procedure, 99
supranormal vision, 12, 43, 44
surface ablation, 66
  see PRK (photorefractive keratectomy)
surgeon personal statistics
  astigmatism, 55
  high hyperopia, 55
  high myopia, 54
  low hyperopia, 54

mild astigmatism, 55
mild myopia, 53
moderate hyperopia, 54
moderate myopia, 54
swimming, surfing, hot tubs, 51, 60, 88, 92, 105
synthetic lens, 5, 7, 21, 22, 25, 95, 96

T

tear drainage canals, 57
tear production, 35, 41, 57
  testing, 69
tear quality, 35
temporary contact lenses, 25, 121
temporary eyeglasses, 121
temporary overcorrection, 56, 77
thin cornea, 39, 60, 63, 67, 73, 85
tonometer, 35
toric lens implant, 7, 16, 97
treatable refractive parameters, 28
twilight anesthesia, 20, 21, 86

U

ultraviolet (UV) light, 60, 71, 98, 103
undercorrection, 56, 76
University of Rochester, 43

V

Valium (diazepam), 29, 46, 70
Vicodin, 72
vision, 1–14
  and light, 2, 3
  measurement, 12–14
  range of vision, 9, 10
  refractive errors, 3–7
vision correction surgeon, personal statistics, 52
vision correction surgery, 15–26
  benefits, 36
  candidates for, 27–31
  costs, 120

financing, 120
  risk factors, 36
  side effects, 28
visual acuity, 12
visual acuity test, 34
visual stability, after PRK, 73
vital signs, 104
vitrectomy, 108

W

wavefront analyzer, 43, 44, 47,
  70
wavefront-guided LASIK, 13, 43,
  53, 58, 119, 121
Williams, David, 43

Y

YAG laser capsulotomy, 108

About the Authors

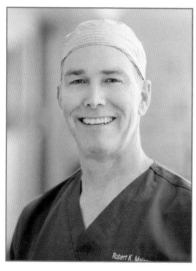

Robert K. Maloney, M.D.,
M.A.(Oxon), is managing partner
of the Maloney-Shamie Vision
Institute in West Los Angeles,
California. Dr. Maloney was
the first eye surgeon in western
North America to perform
LASIK surgery, as part of the
original FDA clinical trials.
Dr. Maloney has trained more
than 1,000 surgeons in the use
of the excimer laser and has
personally performed more
than 65,000 vision correction
surgeries. He was voted by his
peers one of America's top ten
vision correction specialists in
a nationwide survey conducted by *Ophthalmology Times*.

Dr. Maloney is a former Rhodes scholar and *summa cum
laude* graduate of Harvard University. He is the recipient of
the prestigious Lans Distinguished Award, given annually by
the International Society of Refractive Surgery to onesurgeon
in the world for innovative contributions to the field of vision
correction surgery.

Dr. Maloney holds eight patents. He is the author of four
books and more than 175 articles, abstracts, and reports in
professional journals. He has delivered more than 400 lectures
on five continents to professional audiences. He has been a
principal investigator for twenty FDA clinical trials.

Dr. Maloney has appeared frequently on television as the LASIK surgeon for the ABC hit series *Extreme Makeover*. He has appeared on the Discovery Channel, the Learning Channel, NBC, ABC, PBS, and CNN. He has also been featured in numerous magazines and newspapers.

He is married to Nicole Miller Maloney, a photographic artist. They have three children.

Dr. Maloney may be reached by calling the Maloney-Shamie Vision Institute at (310) 208-3937, or he may be reached at the website: **www.maloneyshamie.com.**

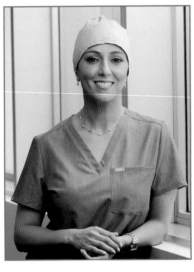

Neda Shamie, M.D., is a renowned LASIK, cataract, and corneal surgeon, and partner of the Maloney-Shamie Vision Institute in West Los Angeles, California. She previously was the medical director of the Doheny Eye Institute and is a clinical professor of ophthalmology at the USC Keck School of Medicine.

Dr. Shamie graduated *summa cum laude* from UCLA and obtained her medical degree from UCSF School of Medicine. She completed her residency and fellowship training in corneal and laser refractive surgery at UC Irvine where she also served as Director of the Corneal Service. Soon thereafter she joined the Devers Eye Institute in Portland, Oregon, where together with Dr. Mark Terry, they spearheaded many projects and advances in the field of lamellar corneal transplantation with emphasis on endothelial keratoplasty (DSEK and DMEK).

Dr. Shamie was the first surgeon in the Northwest to offer both artificial corneal transplantation and DMEK surgery to her patients. Recognized as an expert in complex vision correction surgery, Dr. Shamie has coauthored over fifty publications on the topics of cataract surgery and corneal transplantation, written eight chapters for surgical textbooks, and has led international lectures, courses, and seminars teaching colleagues about the advances in vision correction surgery. In 2017, the American Academy of Ophthalmology awarded her the Senior Achievement Award for contributions to the education of other eye surgeons. She has trained and instructed over 500 surgeons and has personally performed over 6,500 vision correction surgeries.

She is an active member of numerous ophthalmic societies, has served on the Cornea Clinical Committee of the American Society of Cataract and Refractive Surgery, was the president of the Los Angeles Society of Ophthalmology, and has been voted by peers to be among America's Top Doctors.

Dr. Shamie has two young daughters and is married to her college sweetheart, Sia Daneshmand, who is the head of Urologic Oncology at USC. In her spare time, she loves to travel to new destinations and create lasting memories with her family and friends.

Dr. Shamie may be reached by calling the Maloney-Shamie Vision Institute at (310) 208-3937, or she may be reached at the website: **www.maloneyshamie.com.**

Consumer Health Titles from Addicus Books

Visit our online catalog at www.AddicusBooks.com

Bariatric Plastic Surgery	$24.95
Body Contouring Surgery after Weight Loss	$24.95
Cancers of the Mouth and Throat	$19.95
Cataract Surgery	$19.95
Colon & Rectal Cancer, 3rd Edition	$19.95
Coronary Heart Disease	$15.95
Countdown to Baby	$19.95
Diabetic Retinopathy	$19.95
The Courtin Concept: Six Keys to Great Skin at Any Age	$19.95
Elder Care Made Easier	$16.95
Exercising through Your Pregnancy, 2nd Edition	$21.95
Face of the Future: Look Natural, Not Plastic	$19.95
Facial Feminization Surgery	$49.95
LASIK: A Guide to Laser Vision Correction	$19.95
Living with P.C.O.S.: Polycystic Ovarian Syndrome, 2nd Edition	$19.95
Lung Cancer: A Guide to Treatment & Diagnosis, 3rd Edition	$14.95
Macular Degeneration: From Diagnosis to Treatment	$19.95
The New Fibromyalgia Remedy	$19.95
Normal Pressure Hydrocephalus	$19.95
Overcoming Infertility	$19.95
Overcoming Metabolic Syndrome	$19.95
Overcoming Postpartum Depression and Anxiety	$14.95
Overcoming Prescription Drug Addiction, 3rd Edition	$19.95
Overcoming Urinary Incontinence	$19.95
A Patient's Guide to Dental Implants	$14.95
Prostate Cancer: A Patient's Guide to Treatment	$19.95
Sex & the Heart: Erectile Dysfunction's Link to Cardiovascular Disease	$19.95
A Simple Guide to Thyroid Disorders	$19.95
Straight Talk about Breast Cancer—From Diagnosis to Recovery	$19.95

The Stroke Recovery Book, 2nd Edition $19.95
The Type 2 Diabetes Handbook $19.95
Understanding Lumpectomy: A Treatment Guide for Breast Cancer $19.95
Understanding Parkinson's Disease, 2nd Edition $19.95
Understanding Peyronie's Disease. $16.95
Understanding Your Living Will $12.95
A Woman's Guide to Cosmetic Breast Surgery and Body Contouring $21.95
Your Complete Guide to Breast Augmentation & Body Contouring. $21.95
Your Complete Guide to Breast Reduction & Breast Lifts $21.95
Your Complete Guide to Facial Rejuvenation. $21.95
Your Complete Guide to Nose Reshaping. $21.95

To Order Books:
Visit us online at: www.AddicusBooks.com
Call toll-free: (800) 888-4741

For discounts on bulk purchases,
call our Special Sales Department at (402) 330-7493.
Or e-mail us at: info@AddicusBooks.com

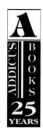

Addicus Books
P. O. Box 45327
Omaha, NE 68145

*Addicus Books is dedicated to publishing consumer health books
that comfort and educate.*